Atlas
and Clinical Reference Guide
for Corneal Topography

Atlas
and Clinical Reference Guide
for Corneal Topography

Editors

Ming Wang, MD, PhD
Clinical Associate Professor of Ophthalmology
University of Tennessee
Director, Wang Vision Cataract & LASIK Center
Nashville, Tennessee

Lance J. Kugler, MD
President and Medical Director, Kugler Vision, P.C
Associate Professor and Director of Refractive Surgery
Truhlsen Eye Institute, University of Nebraska Medical Center
Omaha, Nebraska

Associate Editors

Linda A. Morgan, OD, FAAO
Clinical Investigator and Research Coordinator
Kugler Vision
Omaha, Nebraska

Helen J. Boerman, OD, FAAO
Consultative Optometrist
Cool Springs Eye Care, Franklin, Tennessee
Adjunct Instructor
Indiana University School of Optometry

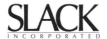

www.Healio.com/books

ISBN: 978-1-61711-027-6

The procedures and practices described in this publication should be implemented in a manner consistent with the professional standards set for the circumstances that apply in each specific situation. Every effort has been made to confirm the accuracy of the information presented and to correctly relate generally accepted practices. The authors, editors, and publisher cannot accept responsibility for errors or exclusions or for the outcome of the material presented herein. There is no expressed or implied warranty of this book or information imparted by it. Care has been taken to ensure that drug selection and dosages are in accordance with currently accepted/recommended practice. Off-label uses of drugs may be discussed. Due to continuing research, changes in government policy and regulations, and various effects of drug reactions and interactions, it is recommended that the reader carefully review all materials and literature provided for each drug, especially those that are new or not frequently used. Some drugs or devices in this publication have clearance for use in a restricted research setting by the Food and Drug and Administration or FDA. Each professional should determine the FDA status of any drug or device prior to use in their practice.

Any review or mention of specific companies or products is not intended as an endorsement by the author or publisher.

SLACK Incorporated uses a review process to evaluate submitted material. Prior to publication, educators or clinicians provide important feedback on the content that we publish. We welcome feedback on this work.

Published by: SLACK Incorporated
                  6900 Grove Road
                  Thorofare, NJ 08086 USA
                  Telephone: 856-848-1000
                  Fax: 856-848-6091
                  www.Healio.com/books

Contact SLACK Incorporated for more information about other books in this field or about the availability of our books from distributors outside the United States.

Library of Congress Cataloging-in-Publication Data

Atlas and clinical reference guide for corneal topography / editors, Ming Wang, Lance J. Kugler ; associate editors, Linda A. Morgan, Helen J. Boerman.
     p. ; cm.
  Includes bibliographical references and index.
  ISBN 978-1-61711-027-6 (paperback : alk. paper)
  I. Wang, Ming X., 1960- editor of compilation. II. Kugler, Lance J., 1975- editor of compilation. III. Morgan, Linda A., editor of compilation. IV. Boerman, Helen J., editor of compilation.
  [DNLM: 1. Corneal Topography--instrumentation--Atlases. 2. Cornea--physiology--Atlases. 3. Corneal Diseases--Atlases. WW 17]
  RE336
  617.7'1900222--dc23
                  2013031015

For permission to reprint material in another publication, contact SLACK Incorporated. Authorization to photocopy items for internal, personal, or academic use is granted by SLACK Incorporated provided that the appropriate fee is paid directly to Copyright Clearance Center. Prior to photocopying items, please contact the Copyright Clearance Center at 222 Rosewood Drive, Danvers, MA 01923 USA; phone: 978-750-8400; website: www.copyright.com; email: info@copyright.com

Printed in the United States of America.

Last digit is print number: 10   9   8   7   6   5   4   3   2   1

Dedication

To our families.

Ming Wang, MD, PhD
Lance J. Kugler, MD
Linda A. Morgan, OD, FAAO
Helen J. Boerman, OD, FAAO

CONTENTS

Acknowledgments

We would like to acknowledge members of both clinic teams that have assisted us in compiling the corneal topographic maps shown in this atlas book and in helping taking care of our patients.

At Wang Vision 3D Cataract & LASIK Center in Nashville, Tennessee, we would like to thank JJ Wang & Drs. Amy Waymire, Meagan Blemker, Gretchen Blemker, Marc Moore, Sarah Connolly, as well as technicians Kayla Sinyard, Scott Haugen, Eric Nesler, Erica Miller, Andrew Langston, Haley Wilson, Ah'lee Manivong, as well as the staff and management at Wang Vision, Ana Martinez, Christin Duncan, Jacqueline Karima, Thomas Bush, Ashley Patty , Suzanne Gentry, Tammy Cardwell, Terry Hagans, Leona Walthorn, and Crystal Micillo.

At KuglerVision in Omaha, Nebraska, we appreciate the effort and support of our doctors, management, and staff: Sheena Blackburn, Kristie Brennen, Patti Fries, Stephanie Gee, Erica Jewitt, Rachel Moyer, Jolene Palmquist, William Schlichtemeier, Anne Silknitter, JoAnn Soukup, Sue Tomanek, Doug Wright, and Jennifer Fischer.

We also appreciate our colleagues across the world who have referred such interesting topographical cases to us for our review and consultation.

Ming Wang, MD, PhD
Lance J. Kugler, MD
Linda A. Morgan, OD, FAAO
Helen J. Boerman, OD, FAAO

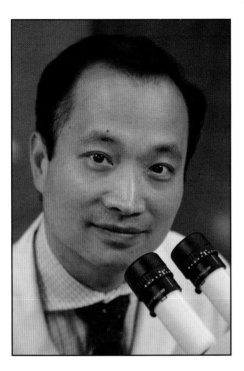

Ming Wang, MD, PhD, is the Director of Wang Vision Cataract and LASIK Center in Nashville, Tennessee, Clinical Associate Professor of the University of Tennessee, and International president of Shanghai Aier Eye Hospital, Shanghai, China. Dr. Wang graduated from Harvard Medical School and Massachusetts Institute of Technology (MD, *magna cum laude*) in Boston, Massachusetts and holds a doctorate degree in laser spectroscopy. He completed his residency at Wills Eye Hospital in Philadelphia, Pennsylvania and his corneal and refractive surgery fellowship at Bascom Palmer Eye Institute, Miami, Florida. He is an editorial board member of *Cataract and Refractive Surgery Today* and *Refractive EyeCare*.

A former panel consultant to the US FDA Ophthalmic Device Panel and a founding director of Vanderbilt Laser Sight Center, Dr. Wang published a paper in the world-renowned journal *Nature*, as well as 5 ophthalmic textbooks *(Corneal Topography in the Wavefront Era; Irregular Astigmatism: Diagnosis and Treatment; Corneal Dystrophy and Degeneration: A Molecular Genetic Approach; Keratoconus and Keratoectasia: Prevention, Diagnosis and Treatment; and Corneal Topography in the Wavefront Era, Second Edition).* Additionally, he has published over 120 papers and book chapters.

Dr. Wang holds several US patents for his inventions of new biotechnologies to restore sight, including an amniotic membrane contact lens, an adaptive infrared retinoscopic device for detecting ocular aberrations, a digital eye bank for virtual clinical trials, phaco balloonplasty, and all-laser no-phaco cataract surgery technology. His invention of the amniotic membrane contact lens has resulted in a commercially available product, AmbioDisk amniotic membrane contact lens, which has been used widely by surgeons worldwide. Dr. Wang is one of the investigators in the United States conducting an FDA-regulated clinical trial to treat presbyopia (Refocus) and to treat keratoconus using cross-linking (Avedro). He introduced the femtosecond laser to China, and performed China's first LASIK procedure using this laser in 2005. He also performed the world's first femtosecond laser-assisted artificial cornea implantation (Alphacor), and the first 3D LASIK procedure. Dr. Wang was a recipient of the Honor Award from The American Academy of Ophthalmology and Lifetime Achievement Award from The Association of Chinese American Physicians. Dr. Wang is a founding president of the Tennessee Chinese Chamber of Commerce, and co-owner and international president of Shanghai Aier Eye Hospitals in Shanghai, China, which is the largest private eye hospital group in China today with 50 locations and holds 10% of China's eye care market.

Dr. Wang specializes in corneal topography, refractive cataract surgery, keratorefractive surgery, corneal and external diseases, keratoconus, and amniotic membrane contact lens. He runs a busy international referral clinic for post-LASIK and post cataract surgery complications. He founded another 501c(3) nonprofit charity, Wang Foundation for Sight Restoration, which has also helped patients from over 40 states in the United States and 55 countries worldwide with all sight restoration surgeries performed free of charge.

Dr. Wang is a champion amateur ballroom dancer and a former finalist in the world ballroom dance championships in the open pro-am international 10 dance. He plays the Chinese violin (er-hu) and accompanied country music legend Dolly Parton on her CD *Those Were the Days*. Dr. Wang organized an annual charity event, a classical ballroom dance—the EyeBall—that is now in its 8th year and has drawn attendees from all over the United States and around the world.

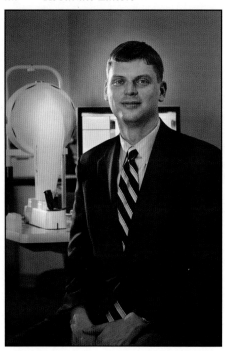

Lance J. Kugler, MD, earned his undergraduate degree from DePauw University in Greencastle, Indiana, where he graduated *magna cum laude* with a degree in computer science. After graduating from Case Western Reserve University School of Medicine in Cleveland, Ohio, he returned to Omaha for residency training in ophthalmology at the University of Nebraska Medical Center. Dr. Kugler then completed a prestigious fellowship in cornea and refractive surgery under the guidance of Ming Wang, MD, PhD, a world renowned ophthalmologist with a PhD in laser physics, in Nashville, Tennessee. Following his year of specialty training, Dr. Kugler returned to private practice and currently serves as president and medical director of Kugler Vision in Omaha, Nebraska where he specializes in refractive and cataract surgery. Dr. Kugler also serves as Assistant Professor and Director of Refractive Surgery for the Truhlsen Eye Institute at the University of Nebraska Medical Center, where he directs resident education and research programs to advance the field of refractive surgery.

Dr. Kugler has authored several peer-reviewed journal articles and textbook chapters, presented at national meetings, and serves as the principal investigator for 2 FDA clinical trials. He teaches several courses at national meetings and also serves as a peer reviewer for refractive surgery journals.

Dr. Kugler has served on the Young Ophthalmologist (YO) info subcommittee of the American Academy of Ophthalmology (AAO) and is a graduate of the prestigious AAO Leadership Development Program.

Dr. Kugler lives with his wife Traci and their 5 children.

ABOUT THE ASSOCIATE EDITORS

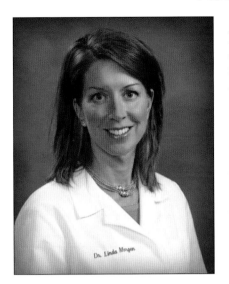

Linda A. Morgan, OD, FAAO, received her Doctorate of Optometry with highest honors from the Pennsylvania College of Optometry in 2000. In 2010, she became a Fellow in the American Academy of Optometry. Her career has included having the roles of Director of Refractive Surgery, Clinical Director, Marketing Director, and adjunct faculty for the University of Missouri, St. Louis. Dr. Morgan has lectured on numerous topics for the optometric community. Currently, in addition to being involved in general patient care, she is a clinical investigator and research coordinator in Omaha, Nebraska, for Kugler Vision. She has been on the Board of the Nebraska Optometric Association (NOA), is past-president of the Eastern Society of the NOA, and is the treasurer for the Optometric Council of Refractive Technology. While also volunteering for the Lions Club and the Special Olympics, Dr. Morgan also spends much of her time with her family and volunteering for the ballet.

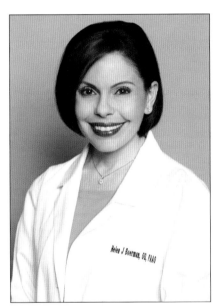

Helen J. Boerman, OD, FAAO, graduated from the State University of New York College of Optometry and completed residency training in Refractive Surgery Management through Indiana University. After completing her residency, she joined Wang Vision Cataract and LASIK Center in Nashville, Tennessee where she served as Director of Clinical Operations, Optometric Residency Director, and adjunct faculty for the Indiana University School of Optometry. During her 10 years of practice there, she edited two topography textbooks with Ming Wang, MD, PhD, and authored numerous book chapters and journal publications on topography, refractive surgery, and anterior segment. She is currently in private practice in Franklin, Tennessee, where she practices consultative optometry, specializing in surgical consultations and post-operative care for laser vision correction, lens replacement, and cataract surgery. She is an active member of the Optometric Council on Refractive Technology and has expertise in ocular surface disease. Dr. Boerman lives in Brentwood, Tennessee with her husband and enjoys travel and spending time with her 2 daughters.

PREFACE

The interpretation of corneal topography has become an important clinical skill for all eye care professionals as our ability to surgically alter the cornea has dramatically improved and patients' visual expectations have risen to unprecedented levels.

Despite advancements in automated indices and reference databases, interpretation of corneal topography remains an exercise in pattern recognition. In the case of pre-LASIK evaluation, for example, there is now a consensus that abnormality in the shape of the cornea preoperatively is perhaps the most important risk factor for the development of post-surgical ectasia. Therefore, understanding the difference between normal topography and abnormal topography has become increasingly important.

However, busy clinicians are challenged to find the time to keep abreast with the latest advances in topographic interpretation. When faced with a corneal topography at chair-side in a busy clinic, one often does not have the time to do in-depth topographic machine-based calculation or go back to the office to pull out a topographic textbook to study the science behind it. There is tremendous value for a clinician to have a topographic atlas book at hand, to quickly compare the clinical topography with maps in the atlas, to identify the clinical condition and formulate the management plan chair-side.

Toward this goal, this atlas and clinical reference to corneal topography has been written.

We believe that eye care professionals will find this atlas to be an indispensable tool, in their daily management of anterior segment diseases at chair-side. If you are reading this in an electronic version, it will allow for chair-side comparison and diagnosis.

We have divided this atlas into three sections:

- In Section I, we review the differences behind the two major types of corneal topographies today, placido-disk topography and elevation-based topography.

- In Section II, we describe a map-based approach to diagnosis and evaluation of corneal diseases. This section is organized by the type of map (axial power, anterior elevation, etc). Maps of normal, disease-free corneas are first presented, followed by maps of the same type in the setting of commonly encountered corneal disorders.

- In Section III, we take a reverse approach and organize the maps based on the disease. In this section, commonly encountered corneal disorders are presented based on their appearance on multiple topography maps.

This book is not intended to be an in-depth manual for a particular topography device, nor a detailed guide for interpretation of automated indices for detection of topographic disease. Such guides already exist and are elegantly written. We feel that there is a need for an atlas of commonly encountered corneal disorders for the busy eye care practitioner.

We believe that all eye care professionals—general ophthalmologists, cataract and refractive surgeons, corneal specialists, optometrists, ophthalmology and optometry residents and fellows—will find this *Atlas and Clinical Reference Guide to Corneal Topography* an indispensable desktop reference, and if you have as an electronic version, a must-have for electronic search, display and comparison at chair-side.

Ming Wang, MD, PhD
Lance J. Kugler, MD
Linda A. Morgan, OD, FAAO
Helen J. Boerman, OD, FAAO

Foreword

Editors Ming Wang, MD, PhD and Lance Kugler, MD, along with their associate editors Linda A. Morgan, OD and Helen J. Boerman, OD, of the *Atlas and Clinical Reference Guide for Corneal Topography* are to be congratulated, with grateful appreciation, for distilling their years of experience and knowledge into this concise and well-organized text. They bring together their clinical understanding of corneal physiology and pathology with topographic images and group them into recognizable patterns. As the first text to use pattern recognition to teach corneal imaging, it introduces a new approach to clinical diagnosis.

This textbook anticipates how clinicians use corneal imaging in practice. Material is provided in two ways. The first uses a *map-based* approach to show how various conditions appear with various imaging modalities, including anterior axial curvature maps, elevation maps (anterior and posterior), and pachymetry maps. The second follows a *disease-based* approach, showing composite views of corneal conditions using the various imaging modalities.

Today's corneal imaging devices have come a long way from the 8-ring Placido-disk systems of the early 1990's, which were limited to topographical maps of the anterior surface and often contained more artifact than information. Today's devices provide a wealth of information about the cornea, and do so using multiple imaging sources, often obtained simultaneously. They minimize artifact using automated image capturing and sophisticated validation algorithms, and even provide diagnostic interpretations, which incorporate information about the anterior and posterior cornea, and corneal thickness.

Most clinicians would agree that corneal imaging has become indispensable to both ophthalmologists and optometrists. Applications are many, and span both clinical and perioperative management. Corneal imaging is used to help diagnose corneal conditions and to assist in fitting contact lenses. It provides valuable information to support IOL power calculations, helps to optimize lens selection, and plays a central role in many refractive surgery decisions. Topography is used to assess the effects of corneal cross-linking and to monitor the progression of corneal diseases.

These applications significantly improve the quality of patient care. At the same time, they present a daunting challenge to the clinician, who must be able to interpret maps quickly and accurately. Different maps may be indicated for different conditions, and knowing which displays to select from the long menus of available options requires familiarity and insight. Being able to differentiate normal maps from abnormal maps—often in the patient's presence—and make important decisions based on the interpretation, requires expertise. Moreover, the fast pace of technological development makes it difficult to stay current with new capabilities.

Corneal images are inherently technical and are often non-specific. The same map might be normal or abnormal depending on the clinical setting. For example, a pachymetry map showing paracentral corneal thickness of 450 microns might suggest keratoconus in a 21 year old but be of little concern in a 65 year old. Central corneal power of 47 Diopters may be expected after hyperopic LASIK but suggest corneal ectasia after a myopic ablation.

These complexities are what make this book so important. The authors use pattern recognition to create associations between corneal conditions and the maps they produce, so clinicians learn to recognize patterns rather than focus on isolated findings. This approach is particularly applicable to progressive corneal conditions, which often present at early stages when they can masquerade as normal variants. The innovative approach used in this book will assist the student and experienced clinician alike.

Pattern recognition is fundamental to everyday life, from the earliest stages of development through the most advanced levels of learning. Infants use pattern recognition when they differentiate between familiar and unfamiliar faces. Master chess players can plan complex strategies after glancing at a chess board, not by studying the locations of individual pieces but by seeing patterns and layouts that are commonly repeated.

Pattern recognition requires familiarity, which we come to recognize as expertise. Experienced automobile drivers come to recognize normal traffic patterns from potential threats in an instant, where new drivers may not. Closer to home, ophthalmologists can readily differentiate an eye that is red from a foreign body from a one with bacterial conjunctivitis, while the difference may not be as obvious to an internist.

Technology is no replacement for clinical interpretation; clinical expertise remains essential. Topography software can use key indices to detect keratoconus but the interpretations are imperfect. Software only uses a small fraction of the total information available, as they can only use information from the current exam. Algorithms cannot place indices in the rich context of a history and other clinical information. In fact, no current technology can recognize patterns better than the human brain, which can identify, evaluate, group, accept and reject cues simultaneously.

The role of the clinician has never been more important, more exciting, or more challenging. The ability to recognize normal and abnormal topography patterns can facilitate clinical diagnosis, and help identify early conditions to prompt timely interventions. Conversely, the failure to recognize a condition can result in untoward outcomes for patients and increase liability risks for clinicians. Even though every eye is unique, diseases follow specific patterns that can be recognized, and learned. As clinicians are called to interpret images across multiple platforms, include hand held devices such as smart phones, the ability to identify topographic patterns will become increasingly important over time.

This book will serve as a standard reference for every clinician who works with the cornea. The innovative organization and systematic approach of this text makes is useful as both a learning tool and a reference. Its value will only increase as the applications of corneal imaging expand in daily practice.

I congratulate the authors on this valuable contribution to the ophthalmic literature!

Guy M. Kezirian, MD, FACS
SurgiVision Consultants, Inc
Scottsdale, Arizona

Section I

Overview of Corneal Topography and Tomography

Introduction to Placido-Disk Topography

Placido-disk topography has been the most commonly used technology since the late 1880s when the Javal-Placido target was developed. Placido-disk topography is based on the reflection of concentric mires (rings) on the cornea. The closer the mires, the steeper the curvature. The wider the mires, the flatter the curvature. Clear surfaces are required for clear reflection of mires. The original Javal-Placido disk devices were never intended to be used a descriptor of corneal shape, but rather were intended to assist in the assessment of corneal optics for refractive correction with spectacles. The application of the placido-disk images were broadened after computerized interpretation of the reflections generated by these disks became a reality in the 1970s.

Placido-disk systems use the reflected image to measure curvature data. Elevation may be calculated by fitting slope data to a predefined mathematical model. This method results in erroneous elevation results and therefore elevation maps derived from placido-disk images will not be discussed in this book.

Wang M, Kugler LJ. *Atlas and Clinical Reference Guide for Corneal Topography* (p 3).
© 2014 SLACK Incorporated.

Introduction to
Elevation-Based Topography

Placido-disk topography has been the standard methodology used for describing the curvature and power of the corneal surface. Placido-disk topography is based on a two dimensional image, however, and is not capable of accurately describing corneal shape. In order to accurately determine corneal shape, a measurement of the Z coordinate, or elevation, is required.

Several systems have been developed over the years to measure the X, Y, and Z coordinates of the cornea in an attempt to determine corneal shape. Of the systems currently available for use, the Pentcam (OCULUS Optikgeräte GmbH) is the most commonly encountered. Due to the advantages that elevation-based topography and tomography hold over placido-disk topography, the Pentacam is rapidly becoming the standard for corneal imaging, particularly when screening candidates for refractive surgery. Due to its popularity we chose to include it in this book, and its images comprise the majority of the images we describe.

The Pentacam uses the Scheimpflug imaging principle, which extends the depth of focus to effectively image the entire anterior segment. The trade-off to this depth of focus is distortion of the image, which the Pentacam corrects via software computation. The Pentacam is a rotating Scheimpflug camera that captures 25 to 50 images during a scan, yielding over 25,000 elevation points per corneal surface.

This technology has several advantages over traditional placido-disk technology. Placido-disk technology uses several assumptions inherent to power calculation. Placido-disk topographers are only capable of measuring the anterior surface, without any input from the posterior surface, thus are unable to measure true corneal power. To overcome this deficiency, placido-disk topographers assume that the posterior surface radius of curvature is 82% of the anterior surface radius of curvature, which leads to significant error particularly in eyes post refractive surgery. The Pentacam, in contrast, directly measures elevation data and therefore true power maps are attainable.

Placido-disk systems also create error by using paracentral measurements and derive peripheral measurements via assumptions. In many corneal conditions, such as prior refractive surgery, the variability of the central cornea relative to the periphery may be substantial.

To ease clinicians' transition from placido-disk topographers to elevation-based tomography, the Pentacam includes an axial power map that is designed to replicate what a placido-disk topographer would measure. This map is derived from the directly measured elevation data, and therefore is prone to the same errors in assumption that occur with any derived maps.

Elevations maps, and the concept of a reference plane, are covered in more detail in Chapter 4.

PACHYMETRIC MAPS

The remaining map on the typical Pentacam four-map view is called the topometric map, or pachymetric map. This map not only determines the central or paracentral corneal thickness, as has been traditionally determined

Wang M, Kugler LJ. *Atlas and Clinical Reference Guide for Corneal Topography (pp 5-6).* © 2014 SLACK Incorporated.

by ultrasound, but it also describes the distribution of the corneal thickness throughout the entire corneal diameter.

Pachymetric data is useful in screening refractive surgery candidates, as it assists in the estimation of residual stromal bed thickness. It also provides invaluable data when ruling out subclinical keratoconus (FFKC), as it distinguishes whether the thinnest point corresponds with the corneal apex.

SECTION II

MAP-BASED APPROACH TO DIAGNOSIS/EVALUATION

3

Axial Curvature Maps

The axial power map is the traditional primary representation of corneal power. The values and colors of each point in an axial power map represent the power associated to a sphere having the same radius of curvature as the cornea at that point. The light refracted at each point is done so with the same power as such a sphere at that point.

The axial power map is a rough descriptor of corneal optics, but does not describe shape. Any representation of shape derived from an axial power map must make assumptions about what shape is required to generate the optics described. At each point in the axial power map, the curvature and height of the centered sphere are not the same as the curvature and height of the cornea. This discrepancy is even more pronounced near the periphery of the map, therefore the shape is distorted.

Despite these shortcomings, the axial power map remains the most commonly encountered topography map and is often the only technology available in a given clinical setting. An axial power map does have some utility as a simple descriptor of corneal astigmatism, including cylinder, axis, and irregularity.

Due to its ubiquity in corneal topographic imaging, the placido disc axial power map is still in use and often is the only technology available in a given clinical setting. Furthermore, many of the classical descriptions of corneal conditions are based on placido-disk images. Therefore we have included it in this book. We chose to use axial power maps from the Zeiss Atlas corneal topographer, as it is one of the most commonly used devices internationally. Axial power maps generated from other devices are similar in appearance, and therefore the same principles in general may be applied.

AXIAL POWER MAPS ON THE OCULUS PENTACAM

This book makes an important distinction between axial power maps generated from elevation based corneal topographers such as the Pentacam (OCULUS Optikgeräte GmbH). The Pentacam directly measures elevation and then derives axial curvature from the elevation data. Because the axial power map is derived indirectly, the accuracy of the axial map is limited. As the resolution, speed, and software of the Pentacam have improved, so have the axial power maps.

Since axial power maps have always been a limited way of viewing the corneal surface and contour, any additional limitations caused by deriving data from elevation data are not likely to be clinically significant. However, it is important to be aware of the relative limitations of any topographical map.

Wang M, Kugler LJ. *Atlas and Clinical Reference Guide for Corneal Topography (pp 9-19).* © 2014 SLACK Incorporated.

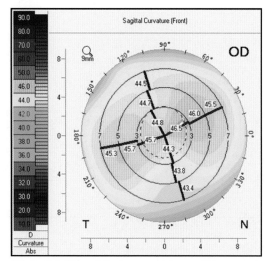

Figure 3-1. Normal Pentacam axial map. This example shows an eye with regular astigmatism, with the steep axis at the 28-degree meridian.

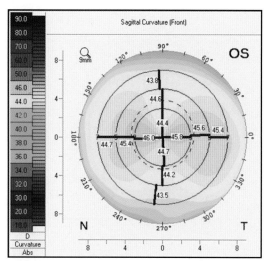

Figure 3-2. Normal Pentacam axial map of an eye with 2.00-diopter (D) cylinder. Another example of a normal Pentacam axial curvature map, with against-the-rule astigmatism.

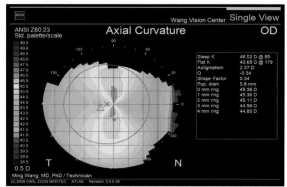

Figure 3-3. Normal Zeiss Atlas map of an eye with moderate astigmatism. This example is from an eye with regular with-the-rule astigmatism of approximately 2.40 D.

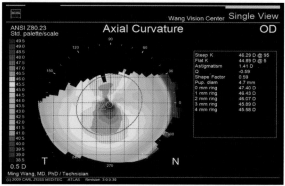

Figure 3-4. Normal Zeiss Atlas map of an eye with moderate astigmatism. This is another example of with-the-rule astigmatism.

AXIAL CURVATURE: KERATOCONUS

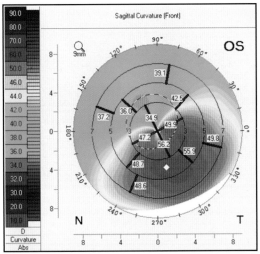

Figure 3-5. This map shows the inferior steepening typical of an eye with keratoconus. Superior nasal flattening is offset by inferior temporal steepening.

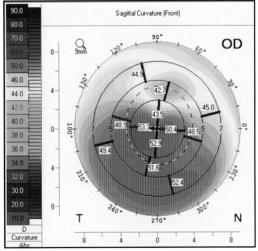

Figure 3-6. Example of the inferior steepening that is typical of the axial curvature maps in patients with keratoconus.

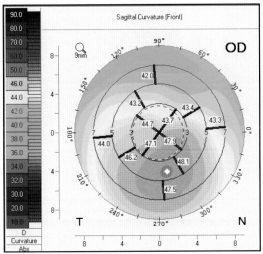

Figure 3-7. Case of mild keratoconus, with the steepest area inferiorly being approximately 48.00 D. The diagnosis of keratoconus would be impossible with keratometry (K) readings alone. Inferior steepening aids in making the diagnosis.

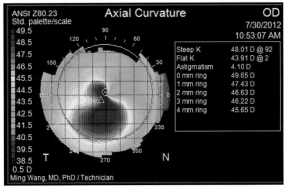

Figure 3-8. An asymmetric bow-tie pattern is shown on Placido-disk topography, which is classically described in early keratoconus patients. This is in contrast to a symmetric bow-tie pattern seen in normal eyes with regular astigmatism (Figure 3-1). This axial curvature map is from the Atlas topographer. The steep K readings are at 48.01 D, as shown in the scale to the right. However, the 0-mm ring shows steep K readings of 49.65 D. This is one example of the importance of reading full mapping instead of only the K readings, which would miss the steepest portion of the cornea.

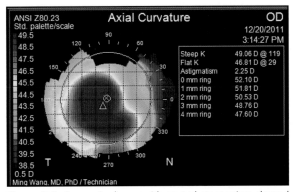

Figure 3-9. An eye is shown with central steepening, skewed inferiorly, which is consistent with keratoconus. This axial curvature map shows K readings of 49.06 and 46.81 D. Again, without looking at the curvature in the individual rings, the K readings appear normal. However, the steepest ring segment shows 52.10 D.

AXIAL CURVATURE: PELLUCID MARGINAL DEGENERATION

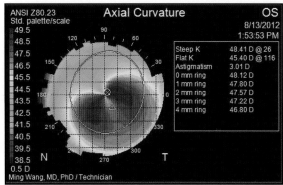

Figure 3-10. Example of a bent bow tie, which is classically associated with pellucid marginal degeneration.

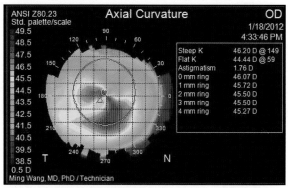

Figure 3-11. An eye is shown with inferior steepening and a bent bow tie, which is associated with pellucid marginal degeneration.

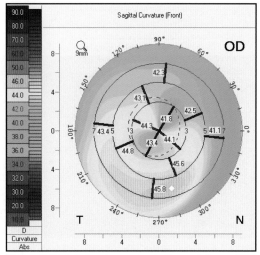

Figure 3-12. Inferior steepening in the periphery of the cornea often associated with pellucid marginal degeneration is shown. This pattern is classically referred to as a "crab claw."

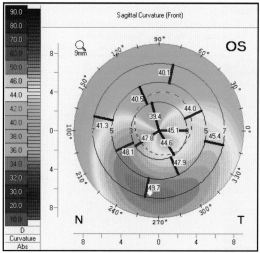

Figure 3-13. Inferior steepening and a bent bow-tie appearance represent pellucid marginal degeneration. The crab-claw appearance is more pronounced in this example.

AXIAL CURVATURE: POST REFRACTIVE SURGERY

Axial Curvature: Post Radial Keratotomy

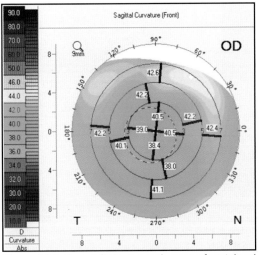

Figure 3-14. Central flattening with areas of peripheral steepening are typical of corneas post radial keratotomy (RK). RK incisions were intended to steepen the midperiphery, resulting in central flattening to correct myopia.

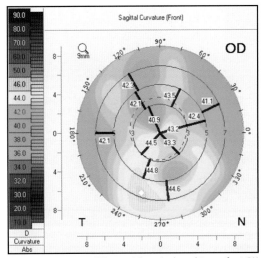

Figure 3-15. A post-RK eye with typical markings of a 4-RK incision cornea is shown. The pattern of inferior steepening with a crab-claw appearance may be confused with pellucid marginal degeneration, but it is due to the RK incisions.

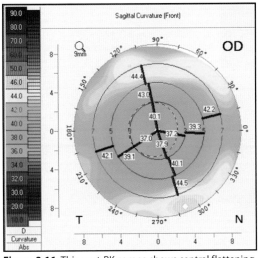

Figure 3-16. This post-RK cornea shows central flattening. The irregularity of the flattening centrally, combined with steepening in the far periphery, is typical of post-RK eyes.

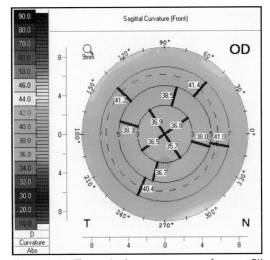

Figure 3-17. The sagittal curvature map of a post-RK patient shows the typical flattening in blue with midperipheral steepening in darker green. Note the irregular pattern of flattening centrally. Eyes after laser-assisted in-situ keratomileusis (LASIK) or photorefractive keratectomy (PRK) also have central flattening, but it is typically much more regular than post-RK eyes.

Axial Curvature: Post Photorefractive Keratectomy

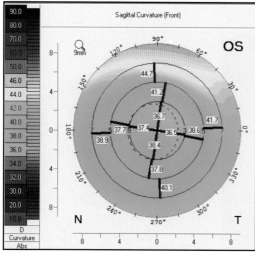

Figure 3-18. This post-PRK axial curvature map shows relatively uniform K readings. Superior steepening represents an area of step-down, which is posterior to the area of central flattening anteriorly. This is a good example demonstrating that axial power maps show curvature and not shape.

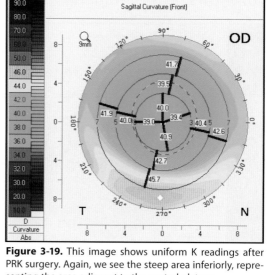

Figure 3-19. This image shows uniform K readings after PRK surgery. Again, we see the steep area inferiorly, representing the area adjacent to the central plateau.

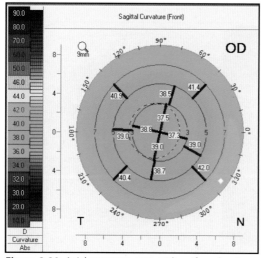

Figure 3-20. Axial curvature map with uniform keratometry readings after PRK.

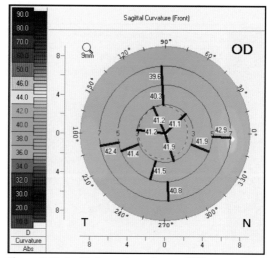

Figure 3-21. Sagittal curvature of a post-PRK cornea showing normal readings. This map is grossly normal, and the fact that this patient had PRK may be easily missed at first glance.

Axial Curvature: Post-LASIK

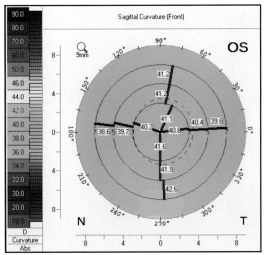

Figure 3-22. This post-LASIK axial curvature map shows some residual with-the-rule astigmatism. Without knowing the patient's history, it would be difficult to determine that this eye is post-LASIK.

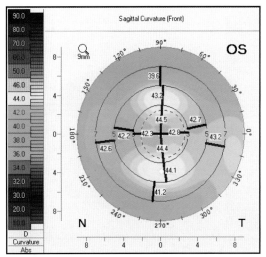

Figure 3-23. This axial curvature map shows a patient post astigmatic LASIK. The optical zone was likely small, resulting in the 2 step-down areas of relative steepening superiorly and inferiorly.

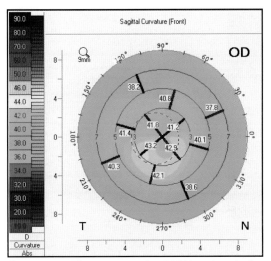

Figure 3-24. This postoperative LASIK patient had a small amount of hyperopia prior to treatment. Note the increased steepening centrally relative to the periphery, which is the hallmark of post hyperopic LASIK. These findings are subtle and may be easily missed.

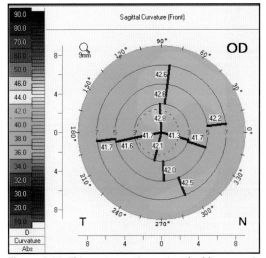

Figure 3-25. This postoperative patient had low myopia prior to surgery. Again, there would not be a way to reliably determine that this eye was post surgery based on this axial power map alone.

Axial Curvature: Post Transplant

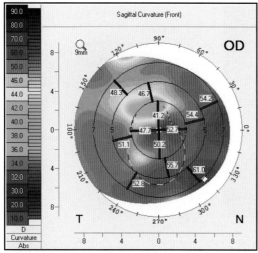

Figure 3-26. This axial curvature map is from an eye with a history of penetrating keratoplasty (PK) surgery. Note the irregularity in topography mirrors the irregular corneal surface that is typical of such eyes.

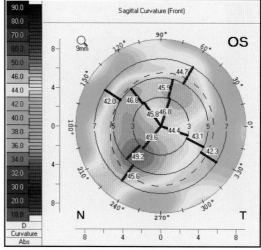

Figure 3-27. Another cornea after PK, with significant irregular astigmatism.

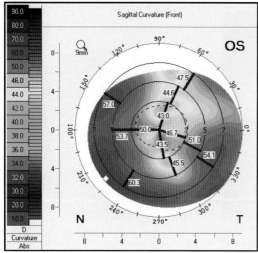

Figure 3-28. An eye after PK.

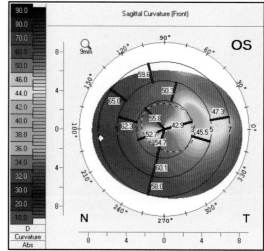

Figure 3-29. An eye after PK, with more than 14.00 D of astigmatism centrally.

Axial Curvature: Post-Intacs Implantation

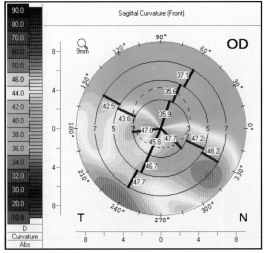

Figure 3-30. This corneal topography clearly shows flattening in the areas of the Intacs (Addition Technology, Inc) ring segments, at the 60- and 240-degree marks.

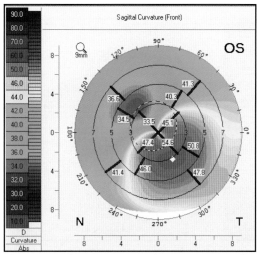

Figure 3-31. This post-Intacs axial curvature map is flatter than the preoperative map. However, this shows the importance of sometimes comparing 2 maps to determine whether a specific treatment is beneficial.

Axial Curvature: Post Conductive Keratoplasty

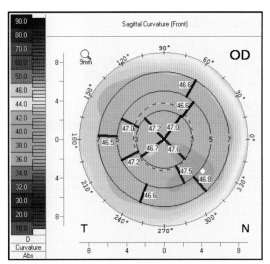

Figure 3-32. Conductive keratoplasty (CK) induces peripheral flattening and central steepening similar to hyperopic LASIK.

AXIAL CURVATURE: IRREGULAR ASTIGMATISM

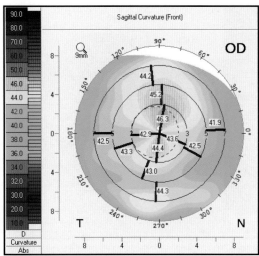

Figure 3-33. Sagittal curvature map showing an eye with irregular astigmatism as the curvature values change across different points on the cornea.

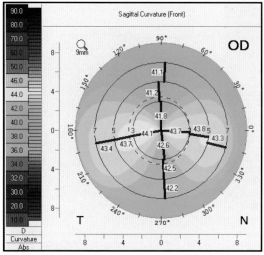

Figure 3-34. Sagittal curvature map of an eye with irregular astigmatism shows how the horizontal meridian changes across the cornea.

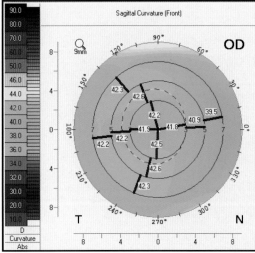

Figure 3-35. Irregular astigmatism can affect the vertical meridians, as shown in this sagittal curvature map. Note that the steep axis (red) is not orthogonal to the flat axis (blue).

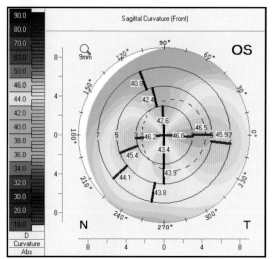

Figure 3-36. Sagittal curvature map showing a change in curvature in both the horizontal and vertical meridians.

AXIAL CURVATURE: POST SURGICAL ECTASIA

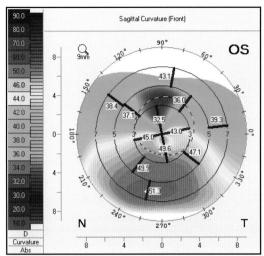

Figure 3-37. Axial curvature map showing an example of post-LASIK ectasia. Without knowing the patient's history, this pattern is not distinguishable from keratoconus.

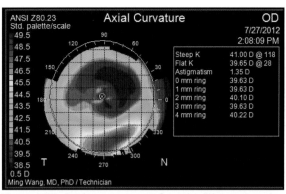

Figure 3-38. Axial curvature map from the Atlas topographer shows post-LASIK ectasia. Without knowing the patient's history, it appears to be similar in appearance to pellucid marginal degeneration. The main clue that this patient had refractive surgery is the relatively symmetric area of flattening superiorly.

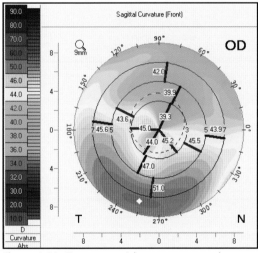

Figure 3-39. Pentacam axial curvature map shows an example of post-LASIK ectasia, with an appearance comparable to pellucid marginal degeneration. Again, this pattern is indistinguishable from keratoconus without knowing the patient's clinical history.

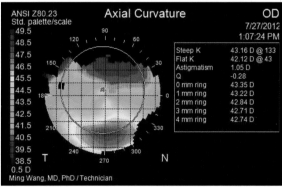

Figure 3-40. Placido-disk axial curvature map of an eye after LASIK. Note that it looks similar to a keratoconus eye with localized inferior steepening.

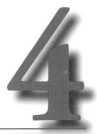

Anterior Elevation Maps

For this book, elevation maps are derived from the Pentacam (OCULUS Optikgeräte GmbH). Elevation maps more accurately describe the corneal surface in terms of X, Y, and Z axes than do Placido-disk axial curvature maps.

The concept of a reference plane may be better understood in the context of a geographical topographic map. Such maps, for example, use sea level as a reference plane. Each peak and valley within the landscape is defined in reference to sea level, with tall mountain ranges appearing red or yellow and deep valleys appearing blue or green.

Anterior elevation maps depict the height of anterior corneal elevations and depressions relative to a computer-generated reference surface. Because the elevation is not based on axis of curvature, this map is a more accurate representation of the shape of the surface and is less susceptible to false-positive findings. For corneal elevation data, the reference plane most commonly used is a sphere with a radius that most closely resembles the overall radius of that specific corneal surface. Such a reference plane is called a *best-fit sphere*. Each point on the cornea is displayed as a color relative to the best-fit sphere. Warm colors, such as orange or red, depict elevations; cool colors, such as blue, show depressions. Although the definition of normal varies, in this book the authors consider anterior elevation to be abnormal if it is greater than +4 μm at the thinnest point or greater than +6 μm at the anterior apex.

Although a sphere is the most commonly used reference plane, other shapes may be used. Another commonly used reference shape is a toric ellipsoid, which is favored by some because of the natural prolate shape of the human cornea. The alignment of the reference sphere may also be specified. Changing the reference sphere for a given cornea greatly changes the appearance of the map; just as changing the sea level would change the appearance of geographical maps. In this book, the authors have chosen to use a best-fit sphere as the reference plane, with a float alignment, which means that the diameter and location of the sphere are chosen to maximize the area of contact between the reference sphere and the cornea.

It is important to remember that elevation maps define shape and not refractive power. Refractive power is not determined by the elevation itself, but rather by changes in elevation. As discussed previously, the refractive power of a cornea is best represented by the axial power map, from which the Pentacam derives the changes in elevation it directly measures. Therefore, although the axial curvature map and the anterior elevation map are related, they do not directly correspond with one another.

Anterior elevation maps are particularly important in refractive surgery. Refractive surgery involves the removal of tissue and reshaping of the cornea, which directly affects the elevation of the corneal surface. It is therefore crucial to understand elevation maps in the context of refractive surgery. For example, with elevation maps it is possible to directly measure the exact amount of tissue removed from a cornea by comparing elevation maps from before and after refractive surgery. Elevation maps are also useful in detecting post surgical abnormalities such as decentered ablations or central islands.

Wang M, Kugler LJ. *Atlas and Clinical Reference Guide for Corneal Topography (pp 21-31).*
© 2014 SLACK Incorporated.

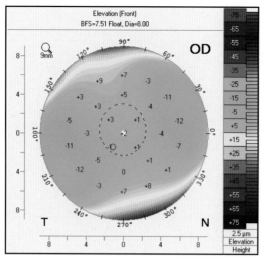

Figure 4-1. Normal elevation map from the Pentacam.

ANTERIOR ELEVATION: KERATOCONUS

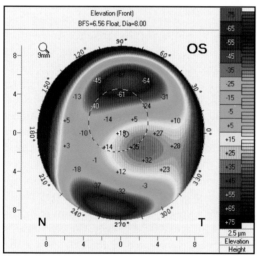

Figure 4-2. Anterior elevation map of a patient with keratoconus shows the typical inferotemporal elevation (red) consistent with the diagnosis. The most anterior elevation is 35 μm, which is well above the limits of normal.

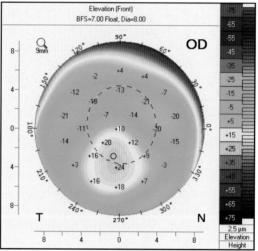

Figure 4-3. Anterior elevation map shows inferior elevation, which is classic for keratoconus or ectasia.

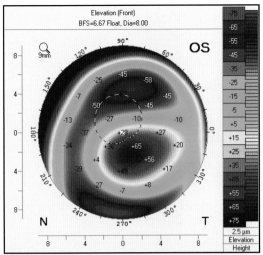

Figure 4-4. Anterior elevation map shows notable inferior elevation (red) of a patient diagnosed with keratoconus.

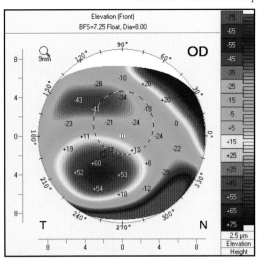

Figure 4-5. The elevation of patients diagnosed with keratoconus is often inferotemporal, as demonstrated in this map. The red area shows marked elevation.

ANTERIOR ELEVATION: PELLUCID MARGINAL DEGENERATION

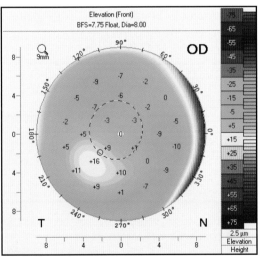

Figure 4-6. The difference between pellucid marginal degeneration and keratoconus is classically demonstrated based on the appearance on the axial power map. Differences in the appearance of the elevation map are minor and are difficult to distinguish from those of keratoconus.

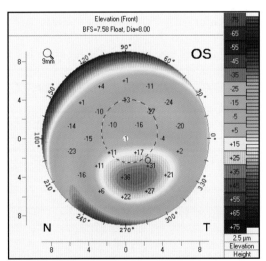

Figure 4-7. Elevation maps show relative elevation from a reference surface. Deviations such as this can appear similar to keratoconus and can be diagnosed as pellucid marginal degeneration only when other characteristics, such as axial power maps, are present.

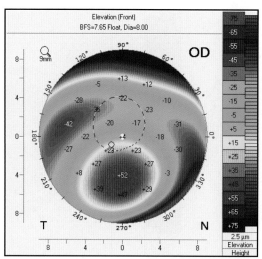

Figure 4-8. Elevation map of a patient diagnosed with pellucid marginal degeneration shows inferior elevation (red). Note that this map is indistinguishable from maps showing keratoconus.

ANTERIOR ELEVATION: POST REFRACTIVE SURGERY

Anterior elevation maps are the most direct way to measure tissue removed by corneal refractive surgery. Anterior elevation maps are useful for diagnosing decentered ablations, central islands, or other abnormal results after laser refractive surgery.

Anterior Elevation: Post Radial Keratotomy

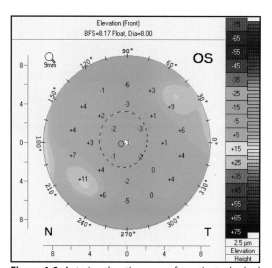

Figure 4-9. Anterior elevation map of a patient who had radial keratotomy (RK) surgery. As with RK surgery, midperipheral elevation coincides with central flattening.

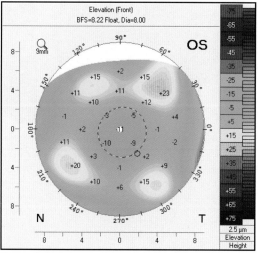

Figure 4-10. It is common to see areas of focal elevation around RK incisions, as the incisions tend to rise anteriorly, relative to the flat central optical zone.

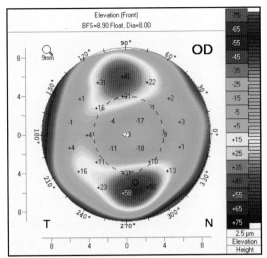

Figure 4-11. Map of a patient who underwent astigmatic keratotomy and RK. The marked elevation in the superior and inferior portions of the cornea corresponds with the astigmatic keratotomy incisions, which have risen anteriorly. Again, the central flattening is the goal of the incisional surgery.

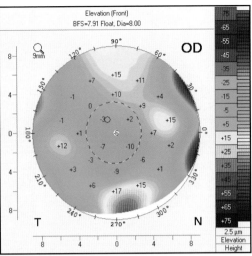

Figure 4-12. Irregularity of the central optical zone suggests the patient may have irregular astigmatism following an RK procedure.

Anterior Elevation: Post Photorefractive Keratectomy

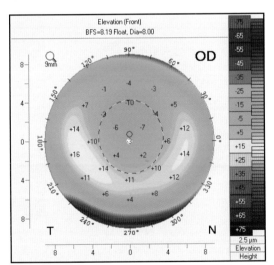

Figure 4-13. Anterior elevation map of a post photorefractive keratectomy (PRK) patient shows significantly decentered PRK ablation. The superior area (darker green) shows the flatter treatment area, which should be over the pupil. The yellow area inferiorly depicts the relative elevation of the inferior midperiphery, relative to the flattened ablation zone superiorly.

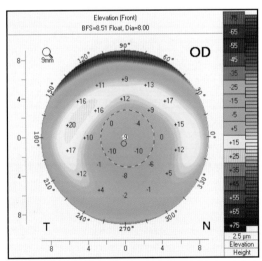

Figure 4-14. Example of a decentered PRK ablation, inferiorly. A crude measurement of the ablation zone suggests the optical zone was approximately 4 mm.

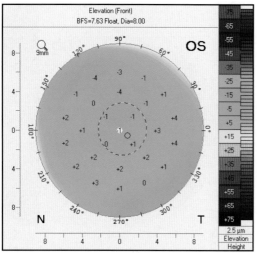

Figure 4-15. Anterior elevation map shows a relatively symmetric post-PRK cornea. Based on this map alone, it would be difficult to detect prior laser surgery.

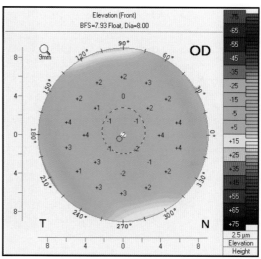

Figure 4-16. Post-PRK anterior elevation map shows elipsoid central depression consistent with an astigmatic PRK treatment.

Anterior Elevation: Post-LASIK

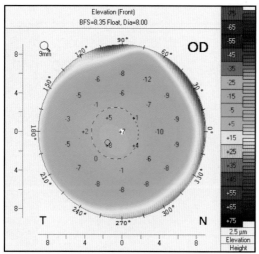

Figure 4-17. Anterior elevation map of a post-laser-assisted in-situ keratomileusis (LASIK) patient shows midperipheral flattening (dark green) with central elevation that is typical of a hyperopic treatment.

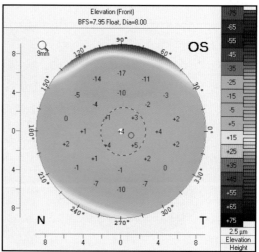

Figure 4-18. Superior and inferior flattening (dark green) shows post against-the-rule myopic astigmatism LASIK treatment in this anterior elevation map.

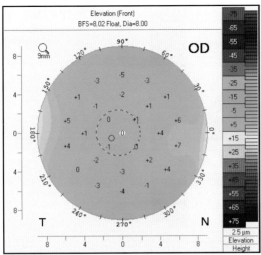

Figure 4-19. Anterior elevation map shows a band of flattening in the 90-degree meridian, which is consistent with a myopic astigmatism LASIK treatment.

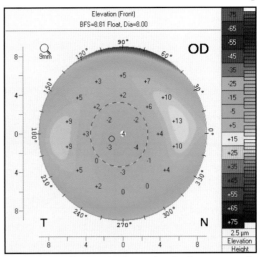

Figure 4-20. Symmetric depression is shown centrally in this anterior elevation map of a post-LASIK myopic treatment.

Anterior Elevation: Post Transplant

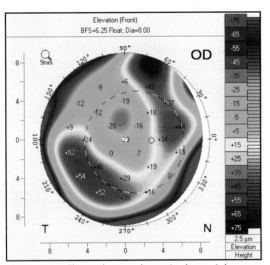

Figure 4-21. Elevated areas shown in the periphery are consistent with the graft-host interface.

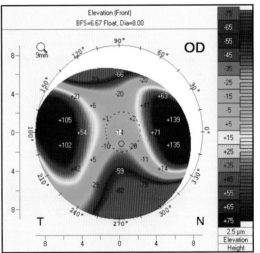

Figure 4-22. Areas of dark red show marked anterior elevation in this map of a patient who had a corneal transplant.

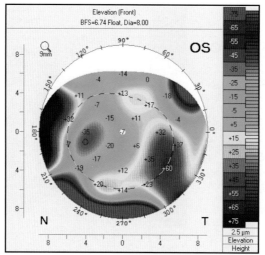

Figure 4-23. A broken suture at the 320-degree meridian is responsible for the elevation shown.

Anterior Elevation: Post-Intacs Implantation

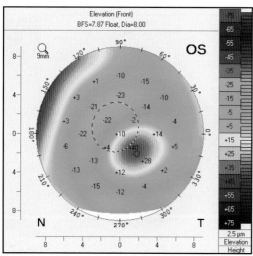

Figure 4-24. Intacs are inserted in the midperipheral cornea. The resultant anterior elevation maps often show midperipheral flattening, as in this eye, which has flattening superiorly and inferiorly to the central cone.

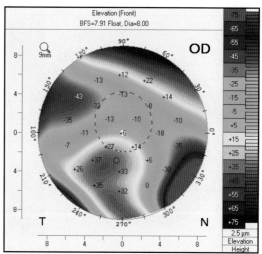

Figure 4-25. Despite the insertion of Intacs rings superiorly and inferiorly, the elevated cone is still present. In this eye, the Intacs achieved flattening superiorly but less so inferiorly.

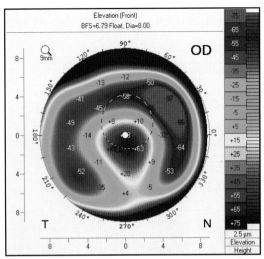

Figure 4-26. The elevated area has been displaced superiorly by the Intacs (Addition Technology, Inc) ring segment inferiorly. Note the significant relative flattening in the periphery circumferentially.

Anterior Elevation: Post Conductive Keratoplasty

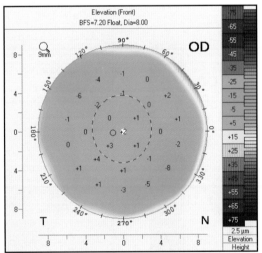

Figure 4-27. Anterior elevation map of a patient after conductive keratoplasty (CK) shows relatively flatter mid-peripheral elevations (dark green), which are often seen with CK treatments. The central area, as expected, is moderately more elevated to enhance the treatment.

ANTERIOR ELEVATION: IRREGULAR ASTIGMATISM

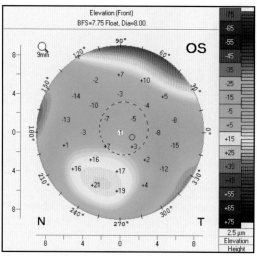

Figure 4-28. The elevated area inferiorly is causing irregular astigmatism in this patient.

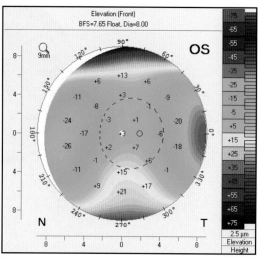

Figure 4-29. Anterior elevation maps of patients with irregular astigmatism do not always mirror the asymmetry of the surface. This map shows a respective hourglass appearance with no hint of asymmetry. Therefore, the source of the irregular astigmatism is likely not to be from the corneal shape.

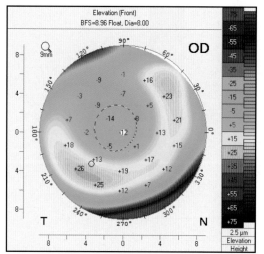

Figure 4-30. The large degree of asymmetry is contributing to irregular astigmatism in this post-LASIK patient with a decentered ablation.

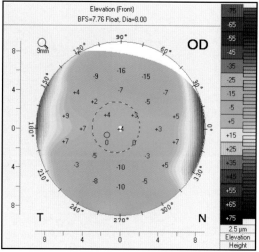

Figure 4-31. Irregular astigmatism cannot always be detected and diagnosed with anterior elevation maps with symmetric findings such as this one.

ANTERIOR ELEVATION: POST SURGICAL ECTASIA

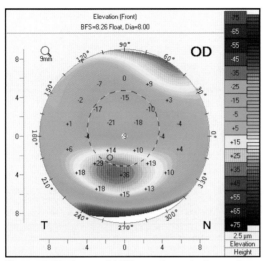

Figure 4-32. A post-LASIK ectasia typically produces inferior elevation with adjacent markedly flat areas of the cornea, as seen in this anterior elevation map in the red and blue areas, respectively.

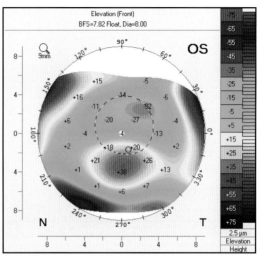

Figure 4-33. Post-LASIK anterior elevation map shows inferior elevation (red) and adjacent flattening, which is often seen in post surgical ectasia.

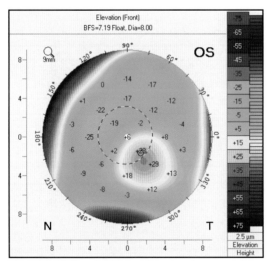

Figure 4-34. Post-LASIK anterior elevation map shows post surgical LASIK ectasia, with inferotemporal elevation and midperipheral flattening.

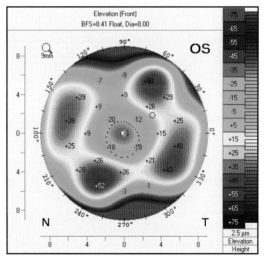

Figure 4-35. Post-RK moderate elevations (red). Midperipheral areas of the cornea are in marked contrast to the central flattening (blue), which corrected the myopia in this post-RK patient.

Posterior Elevation Maps

As discussed in Chapter 2, elevation maps describe the shape of a given corneal surface in relation to a reference plane. Anterior elevation data are particularly important in the context of corneal refractive surgery because tissue is removed from the anterior corneal surface during surgery to achieve the desired contour and power. Although the posterior corneal surface is not directly modified during refractive surgery, posterior elevation data are important in the context of refractive surgery, particularly when screening refractive surgery candidates.

One of the primary goals during consultation with a patient for refractive surgery is detecting the presence of subclinical keratoconus, which is referred to as forme fruste keratoconus. Traditionally, subclinical keratoconus is detected using Placido-disk topography by considering the relative power of the anterior corneal surface. Eyes with keratoconus are known to have increased refractive power inferiorly, relative to the superior portion of the cornea. Various indices have been described to help identify potential cases of subclinical keratoconus, including the commonly used inferior-superior (I-S) difference (discussed in Chapter 3).

Although traditional methods of screening for potential ectatic disease are useful, they are known to have high rates of false-positive and false-negative results. As discussed in Chapter 2, Placido-disk topographers measure the refractive power of the anterior corneal surface, but they do not directly measure the physical shape. Placido-disk topographers are also unable to measure the posterior corneal surface. Keratoconus is a disease process that is first evident in the posterior corneal surface, then it moves anteriorly through the corneal surface until it is evident anteriorly. It is not until the anterior cornea is affected that the disease becomes apparent on Placido-disk topography. Therefore, many cases of subclinical keratoconus are not detected by anterior corneal topography.

Conversely, there are many cases where the power of the anterior corneal surface has an abnormal I-S difference, yet there is no ectatic disease. A common cause of such a false-positive result is due to a cornea that is not perfectly centered when capturing the topographic image. An eye that is looking up may generate a map that appears to have an abnormally high I-S difference, when in fact it does not. In such cases, the posterior elevation map provides useful clues to the normalcy of the cornea. Other corneal diseases may appear as keratoconus on Placido-disk topography, yet they may have normal posterior elevation data. We refer to such cases as *masquerade syndromes* because the condition in question masquerades as keratoconus. These syndromes are described in Chapter 7.

POSTERIOR ELEVATION MAPS

Elevation maps typically relate to the change from corneal elevations and depressions in comparison with a computer-generated reference surface. Elevation maps are more accurate at detecting abnormal corneas, as the elevation is independent of the axis, or orientation, of the corneal curvature. Therefore, false-positive results are not seen with elevation maps.

Posterior elevation maps that have isolated islands or asymmetric patterns may be suspicious for a corneal disorder. Normal values for the posterior surface are ≤ 17 µm and often have symmetric distribution, including an hourglass type of appearance. Deviation > 20 µm is considered an abnormal value. Colors on the map reflect deviations, with red indicating elevations and shades of blue or green indicating depressions.

Wang M, Kugler LJ. *Atlas and Clinical Reference Guide for Corneal Topography* (pp 33-42).
© 2014 SLACK Incorporated.

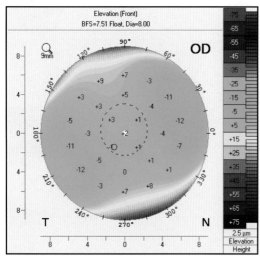

Figure 5-1. Normal posterior elevation map from a Pentacam topographer (OCULUS Optikgeräte GmbH) in an eye with against-the-rule astigmatism.

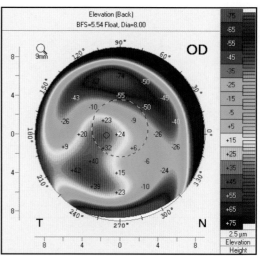

Figure 5-2. The posterior elevation is out of the range of normal. Not only is the elevation increased relative to the best-fit sphere, but the abnormal elevation is inferior in the cornea, suggestive of keratoconus.

Posterior Elevation: Keratoconus

Subtle changes in posterior elevation typically appear on the Pentacam prior to anterior surface changes in early keratoconus patients. If the shape and the location of the curve are outside the normal range and the central 5 mm, the eye may be suspect for keratoconus.

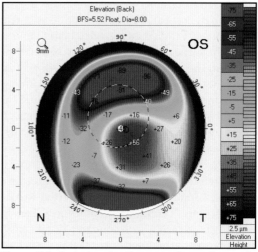

Figure 5-3. Posterior elevation map shows abnormally high elevation inferior to the pupil, which is suggestive of keratoconus.

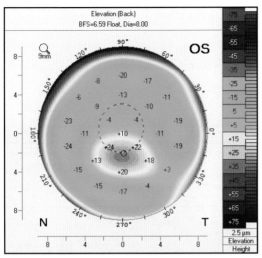

Figure 5-4. Posterior elevation map shows mild elevation often seen in subclinical (forme fruste) keratoconus.

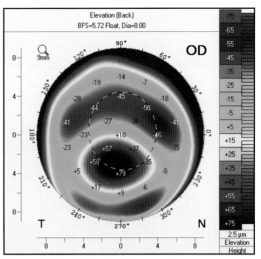

Figure 5-5. Posterior elevation map shows severe elevation in the areas of dark red, inferior to the pupil, which is highly suggestive of keratoconus or other ectatic disease.

POSTERIOR ELEVATION: PELLUCID MARGINAL DEGENERATION

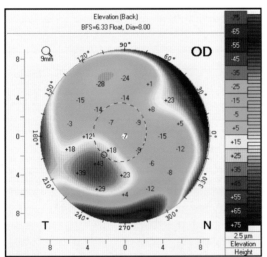

Figure 5-6. Posterior elevation map shows elevation in the midperiphery (area of red). These findings are consistent with pellucid marginal degeneration due to the abnormality in the far periphery.

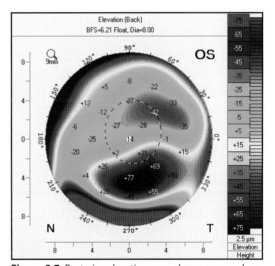

Figure 5-7. Posterior elevation map shows severe elevation in the inferotemporal periphery (dark red). The area in blue shows decreased elevation relative to the reference sphere.

POSTERIOR ELEVATION: POST REFRACTIVE SURGERY

Post refractive surgery does not typically cause a change in the posterior surface of the cornea. Normal elevation values should be found. Any deviation from normal values may indicate ectasia.

Posterior Elevation: Post Radial Keratotomy

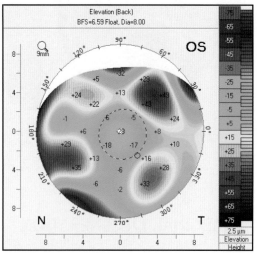

Figure 5-8. Posterior elevation map shows 4 distinct areas of elevation (red areas), which are consistent with radial keratotomy (RK) incisions on the anterior surface.

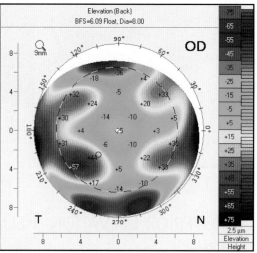

Figure 5-9. Posterior elevation map shows areas of elevation, which are consistent with RK incisions on the anterior surface.

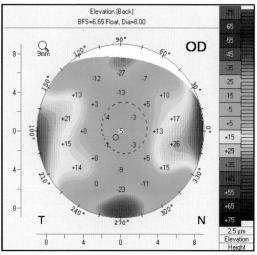

Figure 5-10. Posterior elevation map shows normal symmetry post-RK.

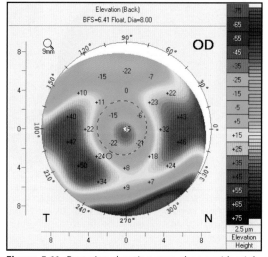

Figure 5-11. Posterior elevation map shows midperipheral elevation (red areas), which is consistent with post-RK patients. Note the central blue area of nontreatment and decreased elevation relative to the reference sphere.

Posterior Elevation: Post Photorefractive Keratectomy

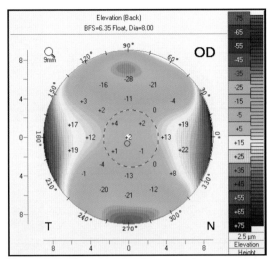

Figure 5-12. Posterior elevation map shows symmetry and no posterior elevation. Because excimer laser surgery removes tissue from the anterior surface, the posterior elevation remains unchanged.

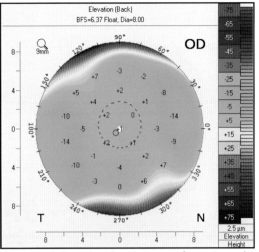

Figure 5-13. Posterior elevation map of a patient who underwent photorefractive keratectomy (PRK) surgery. Elevation is normal.

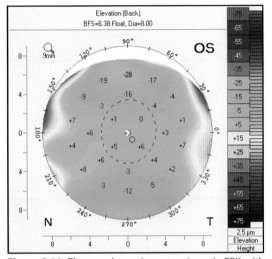

Figure 5-14. The eye shown is post astigmatic PRK with with-the-rule astigmatism. Again, because tissue was removed from the anterior surface, the posterior surface remains grossly unchanged.

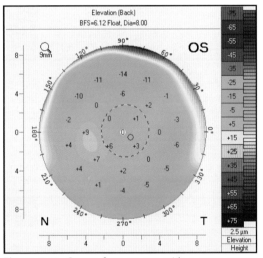

Figure 5-15. Cornea from an eye with a steep cornea before laser-assisted in-situ keratomileusis (LASIK), which has since been flattened. However, the posterior surface remains unchanged.

Posterior Elevation: Post-LASIK

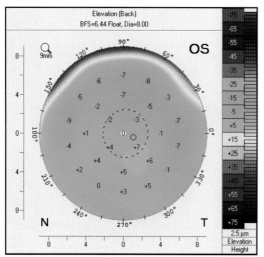

Figure 5-16. Example of post-LASIK surgery posterior elevation map of a patient with against-the-rule astigmatism. The posterior surface should not be altered in LASIK surgery, as is shown in this posterior elevation map.

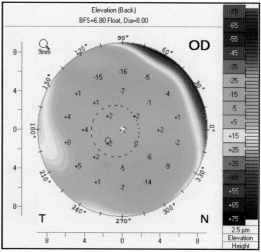

Figure 5-17. Posterior elevation map of an eye with with-the-rule astigmatism post-LASIK.

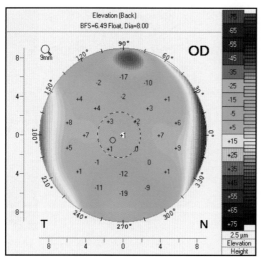

Figure 5-18. Posterior elevation map of an eye with with-the-rule astigmatism post-LASIK.

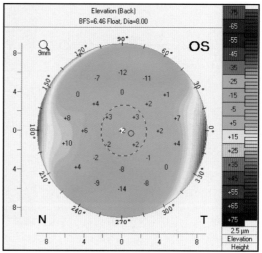

Figure 5-19. Example of a post-LASIK myopic eye.

Posterior Elevation: Post Transplant

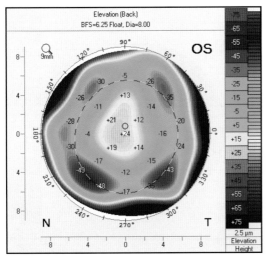

Figure 5-20. Posterior elevation map shows a patient who underwent corneal transplant. The blue areas show decreased elevation, which is consistent with the graft's sutured connection with the recipient's cornea. Relative posterior elevation is indicated centrally.

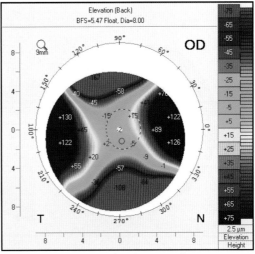

Figure 5-21. Posterior elevation map shows symmetry consistent with high astigmatism.

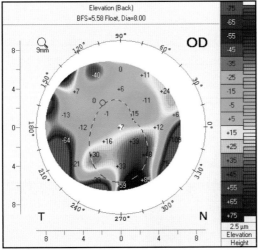

Figure 5-22. Posterior elevation map is irregular and typical of post transplant patients.

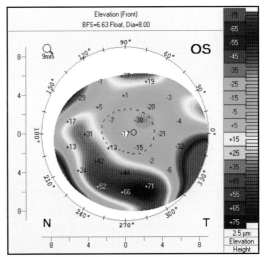

Figure 5-23. Posterior elevation map shows a graft that is decentered superiorly in a patient who underwent corneal transplant. This causes the appearance of relative elevation inferiorly where the graft margin is located.

Posterior Elevation: Post-Intacs Implantation

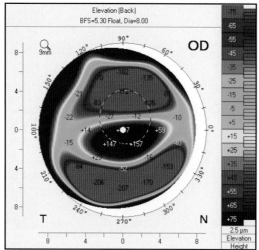

Figure 5-24. Example of a keratoconus patient after Intacs (Addition Technology, Inc) implantation. Posterior elevation, as seen in the central area of dark red, is often noted in patients with keratoconus, even after Intacs surgery, as the Intacs rings exert their effect more on the anterior surface than on the posterior surface.

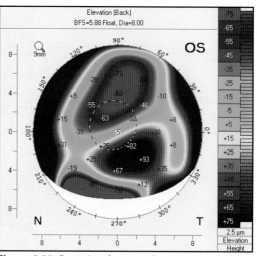

Figure 5-25. Posterior elevation shows severe elevation in the area of dark red inferotemporally, at 93 µm. This patient is post-Intacs implantation for keratoconus.

Posterior Elevation: Post Conductive Keratoplasty

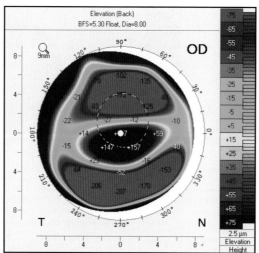

Figure 5-26. Posterior elevation map shows mild elevation centrally with midperipheral flattening in the areas of the conductive keratoplasty spots.

POSTERIOR ELEVATION: IRREGULAR ASTIGMATISM

Irregular astigmatism, by definition, is when the primary meridians of the cornea are not 90 degrees apart, which could be due to corneal warpage after refractive surgery or due to other corneal conditions. Posterior curvature in a patient with irregular astigmatism is typically normal unless it is due to another condition, such as keratoconus or ectasia.

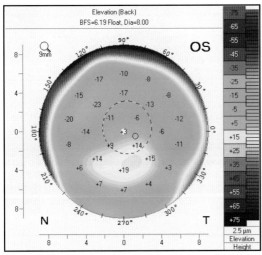

Figure 5-27. Posterior elevation map shows mild inferior elevation in the area of yellow and orange. This elevation is consistent with keratoconus, which is the likely cause of irregular astigmatism in this patient.

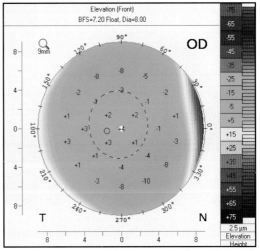

Figure 5-28. Posterior elevation map of a patient with irregular astigmatism. Note that the posterior elevation map is normal. Therefore, the source of the irregularity is elsewhere.

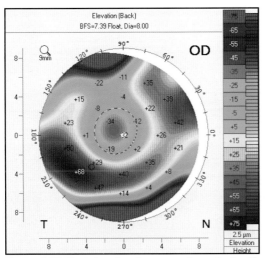

Figure 5-29. Posterior elevation map of a patient with irregular astigmatism after RK.

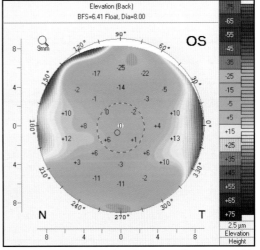

Figure 5-30. Posterior elevation map of a patient with irregular astigmatism. The surface is normal; therefore, the source of the irregularity lies elsewhere and does not arise from subclinical keratoconus.

POSTERIOR ELEVATION: POST SURGICAL ECTASIA

The posterior surface of the cornea does not change after normal LASIK or PRK surgery. If the surface does change, it may indicate ectatic disease. Elevation is typically more than 18 µm and is shown in yellow, orange, or red colors.

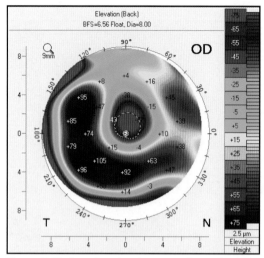

Figure 5-31. Posterior elevation map of a patient who underwent RK surgery and has been diagnosed with post surgical ectasia (area of dark red). The superior central area of purple shows the contrasting flattening, which can occur adjacent to the marked steepening.

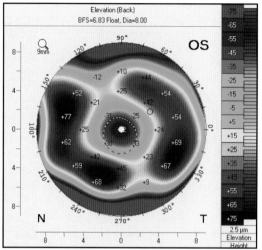

Figure 5-32. Post-RK patient has been diagnosed with post surgical ectasia, which is demonstrated by severe elevation (areas of dark red).

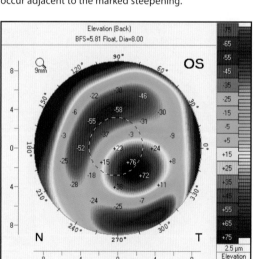

Figure 5-33. Post-LASIK patient was diagnosed with post-surgical ectasia. The difference between the elevations and depressions in this patient is approximately 125 µm.

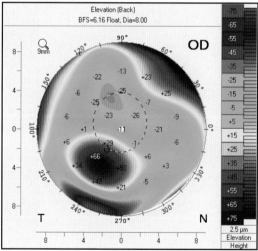

Figure 5-34. Posterior elevation map shows inferior elevation (area of dark red), which is consistent with ectasia.

Pachymetric Maps

Corneal thickness has become an important clinical variable in many disease processes, and it is particularly important in the assessment and planning of corneal refractive surgery. Corneal thickness is also important in the diagnosis and management of corneal endothelial dysfunction, as well as glaucoma. Ultrasound pachymetry has been the standard modality for measurement of corneal thickness since the early 1980s. Despite being accurate and reproducible, ultrasound pachymetry is limited to a single point of measurement, and proper positioning of the probe is operator dependent.

Central corneal thickness is a traditional criterion used for the assessment and planning of refractive surgery. Although the central cornea is the thinnest point in a normal cornea, there are many corneas in which the thinnest point is not in the center. Furthermore, the thinnest value of a normal cornea varies significantly among the population; therefore, it cannot be relied on for the reliable detection of corneal pathology.

The relationship between the central and peripheral cornea can be an indicator of abnormal corneal thinning and may aid in the detection of keratoconus or other ectatic processes. For this reason, the pachymetric maps generated by elevation-based topography are valuable.

PACHYMETRIC MAPS

The pachymetric map is a graphical representation of the thickness distribution through the entire cornea. Pachymetric maps are possible only by using tomography, such as the Pentacam (OCULUS Optikgeräte GmbH), and are not possible with Placido-disk topographers. In fact, the pachymetric map closely resembles the raw data measured by the Pentacam. The accuracy and reliability of the corneal thickness measurements have been found to be comparable to ultrasound pachymetry, which has long been considered the gold standard of corneal thickness measurement. Measurements are displayed on a color-coded map, with red and orange colors representing thinner areas and blue or green colors representing thicker areas of the cornea.

The thinnest area of a normal cornea is within the central 5 degrees and increases in thickness toward the periphery. Normal corneas are thicker in the nasal and superior areas, flattening more temporally. The cornea has a normal central thickness range between 520 and 540 μm.

Findings on the pachymetric map may indicate an abnormal cornea. If the thinnest portion of the cornea is decentered, or the thickness is asymmetric, it may be suggestive of corneal disease such as keratoconus. If the superior and inferior areas of the cornea vary by more than 30 μm, or if the thinnest point varies more than 30 μm compared with the contralateral eye, the cornea may be abnormal.

Wang M, Kugler LJ. *Atlas and Clinical Reference Guide for Corneal Topography* (pp 43-52). © 2014 SLACK Incorporated.

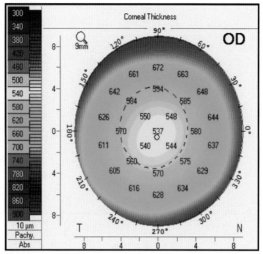

Figure 6-1. Normal corneal thickness map from a Pentacam.

PACHYMETRIC: KERATOCONUS

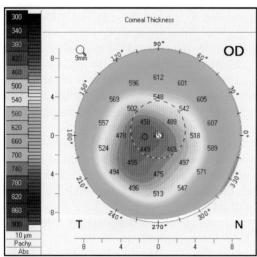

Figure 6-2. The thinnest area of this cornea (indicated in the area of red) is not within the central 5 mm. This appearance is consistent with, although not pathognomonic for, keratoconus.

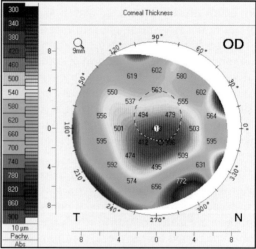

Figure 6-3. Corneal thickness map shows a thinnest point of 396 μm and an irregular thickness distribution pattern. These findings are consistent with keratoconus, which often presents with a distorted cornea.

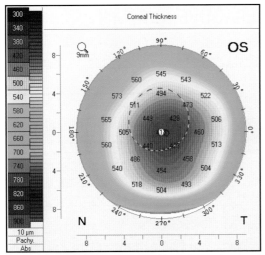

Figure 6-4. The oblong shape in this pachymetric map of a keratoconus patient mirrors the elongated cone shape seen in a keratoconic cornea.

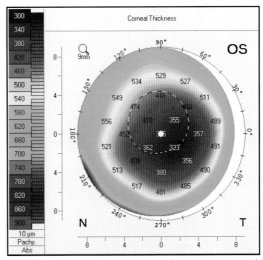

Figure 6-5. Classic keratoconic pachymetric map, with severe thinning in the area of dark red at 323 µm, demonstrating inferotemporal asymmetry.

PACHYMETRIC: PELLUCID MARGINAL DEGENERATION

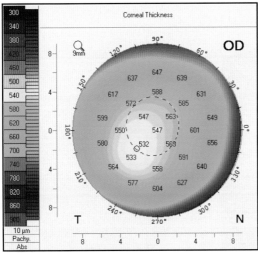

Figure 6-6. This pachymetric map shows inferotemporal displacement of the thinnest point, which is consistent with pellucid marginal degeneration. Keratoconus and pellucid marginal degeneration are generally indistinguishable in a pachymetric map.

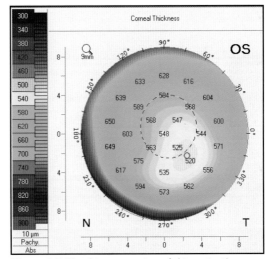

Figure 6-7. The thinnest portion of this patient's cornea is inferotemporal, corresponding to the area of thinning typically seen in pellucid marginal degeneration patients.

PACHYMETRIC: POST REFRACTIVE SURGERY

Pachymetric Maps: Post Radial Keratotomy

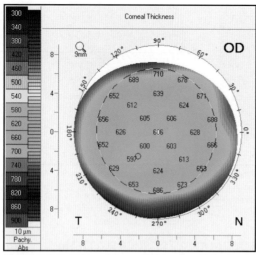

Figure 6-8. Radial keratotomy (RK) involves flattening of the central cornea without removing any tissue. Therefore, the corneal thickness remains in the normal range centrally.

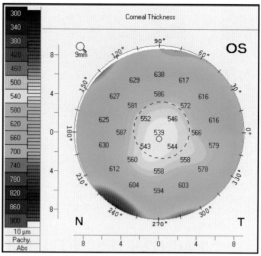

Figure 6-9. Grossly normal pachymetry map. However, there is a hint of asymmetry, which is consistent with a history of 4 RK incisions.

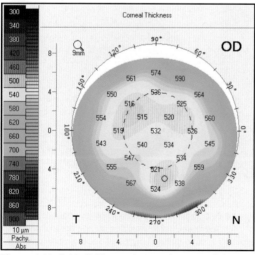

Figure 6-10. Epithelial hyperplasia in the areas of the incisions may lead to increased thickness measurements in the midperiphery.

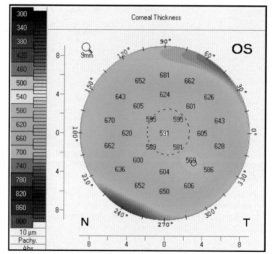

Figure 6-11. A pachymetry map shows a cloverleaf pattern in the areas of light green, which are associated with RK incisions.

Pachymetric: Post Photorefractive Keratectomy

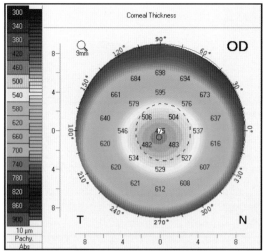

Figure 6-12. Pachymetric maps in post photorefractive keratectomy (PRK) eyes typically have a symmetric area of flattening centrally, with a rapid change in thickness in the midperiphery beyond the optical zone.

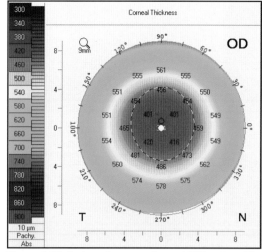

Figure 6-13. Pachymetry map of a post-PRK patient. The large area in red indicates that a large area was treated with PRK.

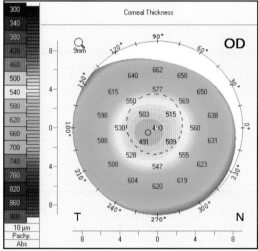

Figure 6-14. Post-PRK corneal thickness map shows a symmetric distribution across the cornea.

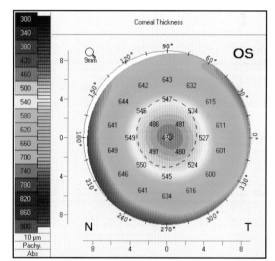

Figure 6-15. Example of a normal pachymetry map of a post-PRK patient. The thinnest area in red is central with uniform thickening within the optical zone.

Pachymetric: Post-LASIK

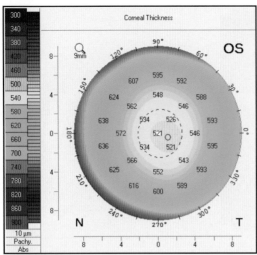

Figure 6-16. Corneal thickness map shows uniform thickness but the center is thinner relative to the periphery. This patient is post-myopic laser-assisted in-situ keratomileusis (LASIK), although this is difficult to determine based solely on this pachymetric map.

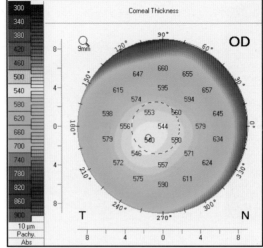

Figure 6-17. This patient underwent LASIK surgery for hyperopia. Note the relative thinning in the midperiphery, which is consistent with the hyperopic ablation pattern. There is a slight decentration of the thinnest point relative to the pupil that is consistent with angle-kappa, which is common in hyperopic eyes.

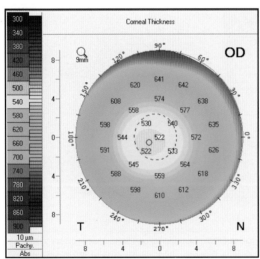

Figure 6-18. Example of a pachymetric map post myopic LASIK.

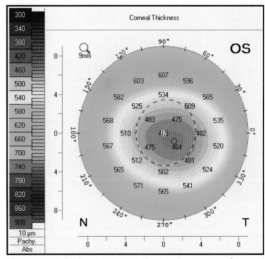

Figure 6-19. Pachymetric map shows a large area of central thinning, which is consistent with post myopic LASIK.

Pachymetric: Post Transplant

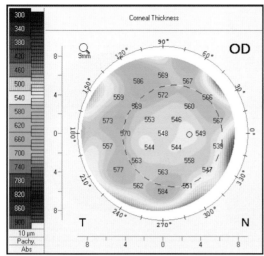

Figure 6-20. Due to the high variability of edema within a corneal graft, pachymetric maps of post transplant eyes are typically irregular with a highly variable pattern. This example shows a relatively symmetric map, with areas of relative flattening that correspond to interrupted sutures in the periphery.

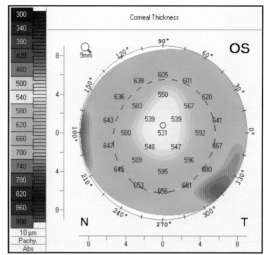

Figure 6-21. Corneal thickness of a well-centered corneal graft is shown, with a relatively normal thickness distribution.

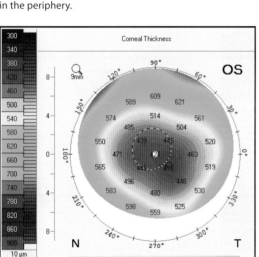

Figure 6-22. The thickness of this corneal graft is below average. This map is indistinguishable from that of a post-myopic LASIK eye.

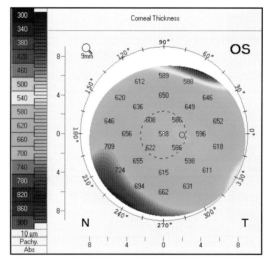

Figure 6-23. The thickness of this graft is above average, which is suggestive of corneal edema.

Pachymetric: Post-Intacs Implantation

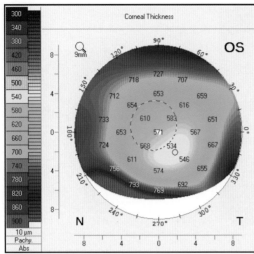

Figure 6-24. The implanted Intacs (Addition Technology, Inc) rings increase corneal thickness in the midperiphery. This map shows a pachymetric progression larger than normal, as the thickening into the periphery occurs at a faster rate due to the presence of the Intacs rings.

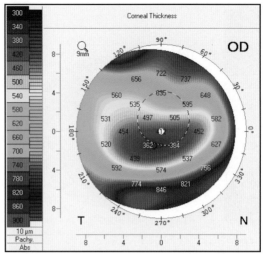

Figure 6-25. This map is from a patient who underwent Intacs implantation for keratoconus. The thin central cornea, measuring 362 µm, is consistent with keratoconus. The thick midperiphery, approximately 575 µm, is atypical of keratoconus, but it is consistent with the presence of Intacs rings.

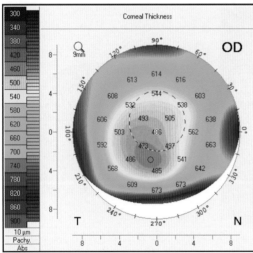

Figure 6-26. Example of an eye with Intacs, which was implanted to treat keratoconus. Marked central thinning, with thickening in the midperiphery, is seen.

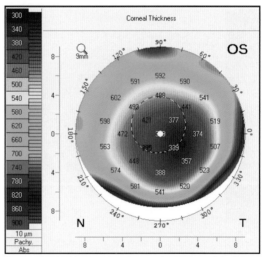

Figure 6-27. This keratoconus eye has severe thinning at the apex of the cone. The abrupt jump from thickness in the high 300 to mid 500 µm range confirms the presence of Intacs rings.

PACHYMETRIC: IRREGULAR ASTIGMATISM

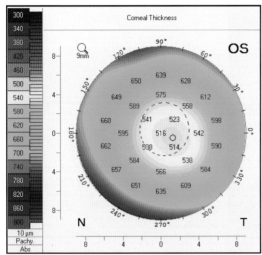

Figure 6-28. Pachymetry maps of patients with irregular astigmatism are often normal, with central thin areas, and progressively thickening into the periphery.

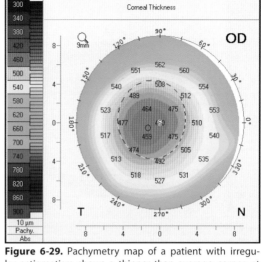

Figure 6-29. Pachymetry map of a patient with irregular astigmatism shows a thinner than average cornea at 459 µm. Without topography or anterior curvature, the diagnosis of irregular astigmatism is difficult to determine.

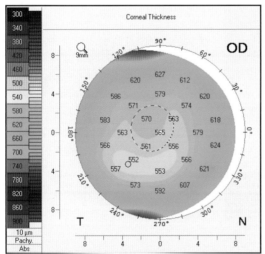

Figure 6-30. Pachymetry map of a patient with irregular astigmatism shows some asymmetry, with the light green inferior midperiphery approximately 25 µm thinner than the superior area, which may account for irregular astigmatism.

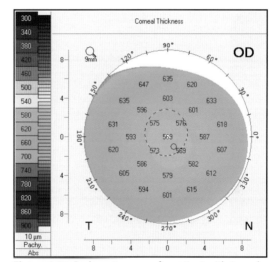

Figure 6-31. Pachymetry map of a patient with irregular astigmatism shows normal corneal thickness and normal distribution.

PACHYMETRIC: POST SURGICAL ECTASIA

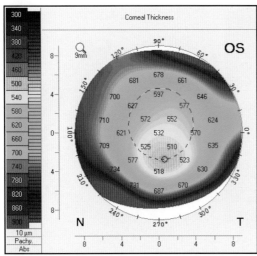

Figure 6-32. Inferior displacement of the thinnest point is shown, which is consistent with keratoconus or post refractive surgery ectasia.

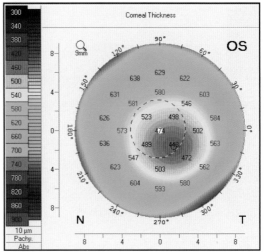

Figure 6-33. Map of a post-LASIK patient who was diagnosed clinically with post refractive surgery ectasia. This pachymetric map is suggestive of either a decentered ablation or ectasia.

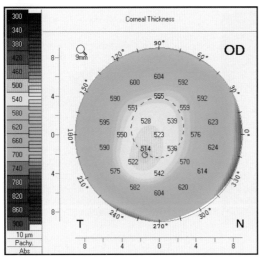

Figure 6-34. The inferiorly displaced area of thinning is consistent with post-LASIK ectasia. Again, this pattern is indistinguishable from keratoconus without obtaining a clinical history.

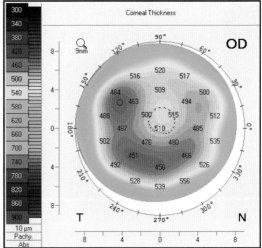

Figure 6-35. Post-RK eye with areas of scarring inferiorly that correspond with the RK incisions. The scars cause erroneous measurement of corneal thickness. The true thickness is much thicker than that represented here. As with any diagnostic test or measurement, clinical correlation is essential.

SECTION III

DISEASE-BASED APPROACH

Keratoconus

In this section, each disease state will be briefly described. Full maps will show the importance of reading all of the maps together to determine a diagnosis.

Keratoconus is a bilateral, noninflammatory degeneration of the eye characterized by paracentral corneal ectasia and steepening, high keratometry values, and often against-the-rule astigmatism. The thinning is reported to originate in the stroma of the cornea.

The prevalence of keratoconus in the general population is reported to be approximately 1 in 2000 patients. Keratoconus has been suspected of being a hereditary disorder, and having a family history presents a significant risk factor for individuals; but dominant, recessive, and irregular transmission have all occurred. This condition has several possible associated risk factors, including systemic conditions, such as Down syndrome, and connective tissue disorders, such as Ehlers-Danlos syndrome. Keratoconus is also associated with other ocular disorders, such as retinitis pigmentosa, microcornea, aniridia, and ectopia lentis. Extensive research into the relationship of keratoconus and atopic disease has been conducted, and eye rubbing can be a precipitating factor in the evolution of the disease. Although a bilateral entity, keratoconus often presents with more pronunciation in one eye than in the other, as well as having an asymmetric and variable progression. Keratoconus usually presents during the second decade of life and typically does not progress later than 40 years of age.

AXIAL CURVATURE: ANTERIOR

Early keratoconus presents on topography as inferior or central steepening, with or without a difference compared with the fellow eye. Mild astigmatism may be present. Several indices have been developed to differentiate these eyes from normal eyes, such as the inferior-superior (I-S) difference, but a high false-positive rate exists. Although these indices may be helpful, the diagnosis remains largely dependent on pattern recognition on the part of the clinician. To that end, in this section we present several examples of eyes with various degrees of keratoconus.

Wang M, Kugler LJ. *Atlas and Clinical Reference Guide for Corneal Topography (pp 55-67).*
© 2014 SLACK Incorporated.

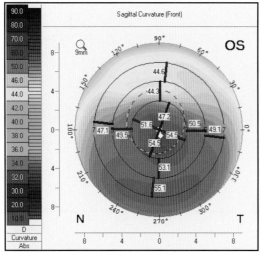

Figure 7-1. A sagittal curvature map shows steepening in the inferior portion of 55.10 diopters (D). This is an approximate difference of 11.00 D from the superior portion of the cornea, which is typical of a keratoconus patient.

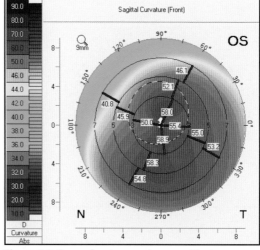

Figure 7-2. Severe keratoconus is seen with steep curvature throughout the central and inferior cornea.

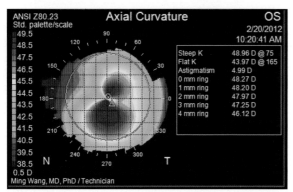

Figure 7-3. Axial curvature map from the Atlas topographer (Carl Zeiss Meditec) shows a classic asymmetric bow-tie appearance, with the inferior loop being larger than the superior loop. Also a slight bend in the bow tie is noted, which is consistent with keratoconus.

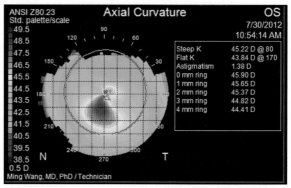

Figure 7-4. A mild case of keratoconus is shown, with obvious inferior steepening and asymmetric bow-tie appearance.

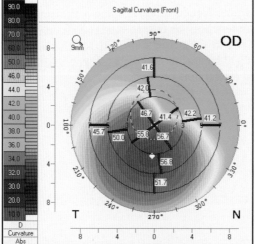

Figure 7-5. Sagittal curvature map shows inferior steepening of 56.88 D, in a classic appearance of advanced keratoconus.

ANTERIOR ELEVATION

As described previously, keratoconus is a disease that progresses anteriorly through the cornea, starting at the posterior surface and progressing toward the anterior surface. Therefore, the anterior elevation map appearance is similar to that of the posterior surface, but this is seen later in the disease process. Although the definition of normal varies, in this book the authors consider anterior elevation to be abnormal if it is > +4 µm at the thinnest point or > +6 µm at the anterior apex.

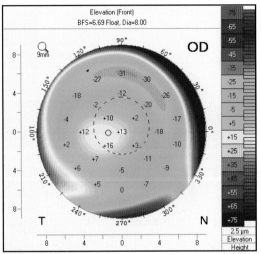

Figure 7-6. Anterior elevation map of a patient with keratoconus shows midperipheral superior flattening and relative elevation (yellow).

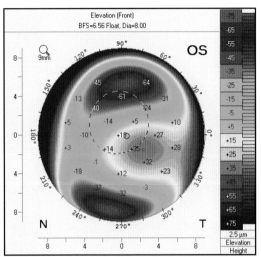

Figure 7-7. The tongue pattern of this anterior elevation map of a patient with keratoconus shows inferior temporal steepening.

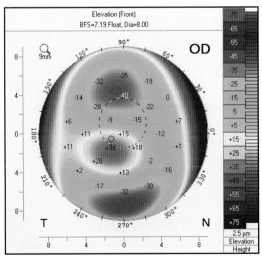

Figure 7-8. Anterior elevation map shows anterior elevation (red), which is typical of keratoconus. The depressed areas (blue) superiorly and inferiorly are contrasted to the area of elevation centrally.

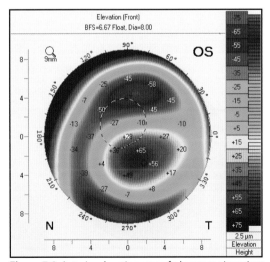

Figure 7-9. Anterior elevation map of a keratoconic patient shows marked inferior temporal elevation (area of dark red) of 65 µm.

POSTERIOR ELEVATION

Keratoconus is a disease process that is first evident in the posterior corneal surface; it then moves anteriorly through the corneal surface until it is evident anteriorly. Therefore, posterior elevation maps are useful in detecting the earliest cases of subclinical keratoconus. As with ante-rior elevation maps, the authors have chosen to use a best-fit-sphere as the reference surface in this book. Although the definition of normal varies, in general, the authors consider posterior elevation of > +19 μm at the thinnest point or > +6 μm at the posterior apex to be abnormal.

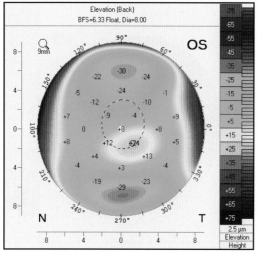

Figure 7-10. Posterior elevation maps are excellent sources of early changes in keratoconic eyes because ectatic changes are first detected posteriorly. This map shows mild elevation in the posterior surface of the cornea.

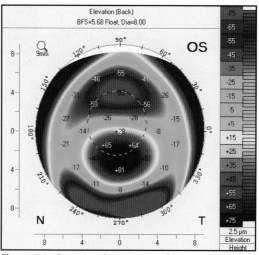

Figure 7-11. Posterior elevation map shows an elevation of 81 μm, which is typical of severe keratoconus.

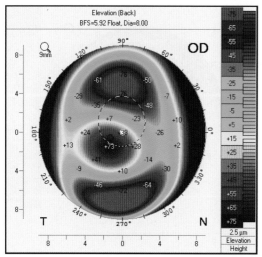

Figure 7-12. The posterior steepening in this map is 73 μm, representing a severe elevation abnormality.

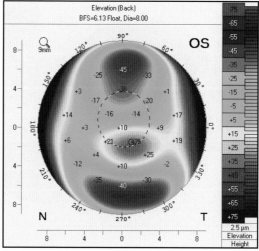

Figure 7-13. The elevation height in this image is of early keratoconus (at 35 μm).

PACHYMETRIC MAPS

Appearance of Pachymetric Maps in Eyes With Keratoconus

Eyes with keratoconus, or subclinical keratoconus, typically have thinner corneas than normal eyes. Keratoconic eyes also have a more progressive increase in corneal thickness from the center to the periphery. In other words, there is a more rapid increase in thickness when moving from the center to the periphery in eyes with keratoconus than there is in normal eyes. Furthermore, the thinnest point of a keratoconic eye typically is inferior to the center of the cornea, which is known as inferior displacement. The pachymetric map on the Pentacam (OCULUS Optikgeräte GmbH) is useful to detect these differences in eyes with possible keratoconus.

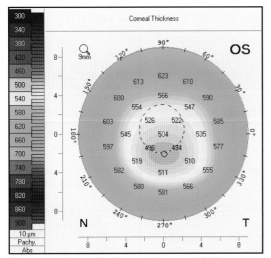

Figure 7-14. Example of a typical corneal thickness map with off-axis thinning, which is suspicious for early keratoconus.

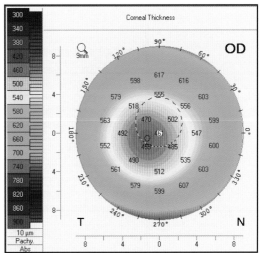

Figure 7-15. Compared with an average corneal thickness of 530 μm, this corneal thickness map is unusually thin at 455 μm.

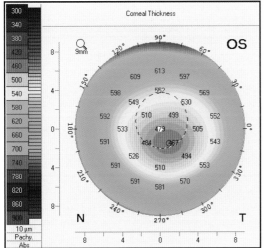

Figure 7-16. Example of corneal thinning, with mild inferior displacement.

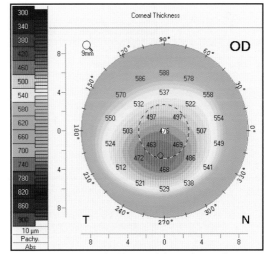

Figure 7-17. As can be detected from this pachymetric map, the rings showing the different thicknesses are also skewed into an oblong pattern, which is often associated with keratoconic corneas. The inferior displacement is also characteristic of keratoconus.

FOUR-MAP REFRACTIVE VIEW

The Pentacam offers the ability to view measured tomographic data in many different formats, depending on the needs of the clinician. The four-map view is the "standard" view of the Pentacam. The four-map refractive view presents 4 maps that are most useful to clinicians screening patients for refractive surgery. This view is useful because it shows the traditional axial power map, anterior elevation map, posterior elevation map, and pachymetric map. Each map provides valuable data regarding the health and structure of the cornea. When viewed together as a group, a tremendous amount of data are available to the clinician on one page.

Figure 7-18. A classic example of early keratoconus is shown. Early posterior elevation can be seen, which precedes changes on the anterior surface. Inferior steepening is seen in the inferior portion of the sagittal curvature map.

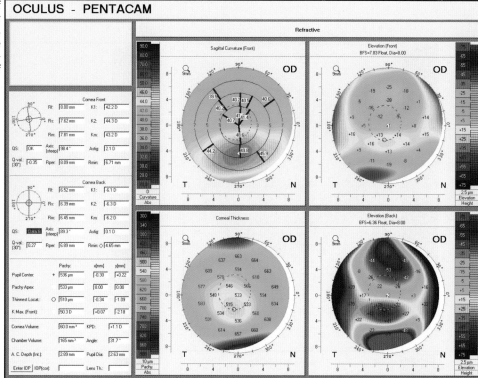

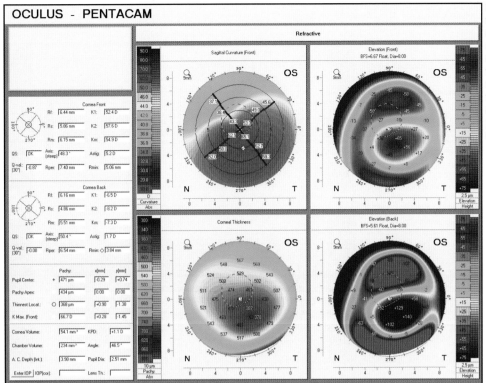

Figure 7-19. This 4-map refractive picture shows an example of advanced keratoconus, with the steepest portion of the cornea at 65.10 D. The corneal thickness and front and back elevation maps show corresponding areas respective to the cone. When these areas correspond on the elevation and pachymetric maps, the authors designate it as "3-point touch."

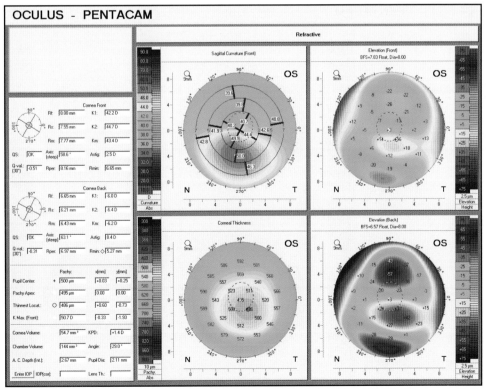

Figure 7-20. This 4-map refractive picture notes that the curvature of the front surface does not correspond with the other 3 maps, which is typical of the keratoconic disease processes. The sagittal curvature is a power map representing the curvature induced by the area of elevation, whereas the remaining 3 maps better correspond with the location of the disease, which in this case is in the inferior temporal area of the cornea.

Figure 7-21. The location of the abnormality in this eye is more central than typical keratoconus. However, the thinnest area of 455 µm, with corresponding posterior steepening and a steepest keratometry reading of 55.30 D, is combined to be diagnosed with keratoconus.

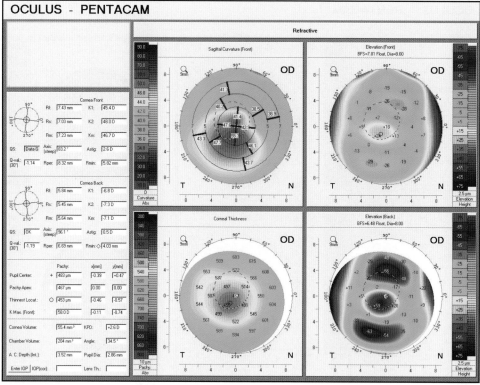

Figure 7-22. Classic example of 3-point touch in an eye with keratoconus.

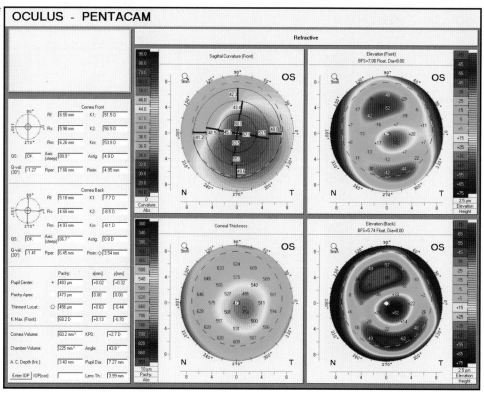

MASQUERADE SYNDROME

Masquerade syndrome is the term the authors have given to corneal conditions that appear to be keratoconus or keratoectasia on topography when, in fact, they are not. This euphemism suggests that these conditions are masquerading as keratoconus. These conditions demonstrate the power of looking at corneas using several different views, or maps, to better define the shape. Each masquerade syndrome may be revealed as a false-positive case of keratoconus by using the 4-map view.

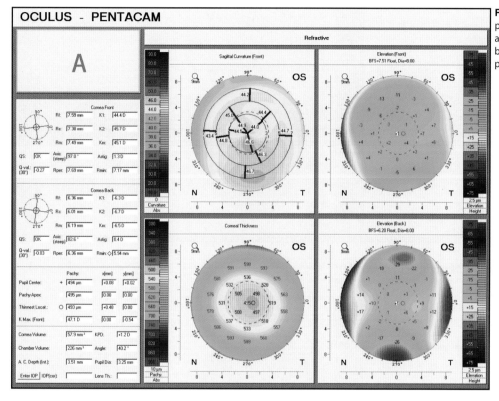

Figure 7-22. (A) This patient's preoperative topographic scans appear with a > 2.00-D difference between the superior and inferior portions of the cornea.

Figure 7-22. (B) After using preservative-free artificial tears for 1 month, the cornea appears normal.

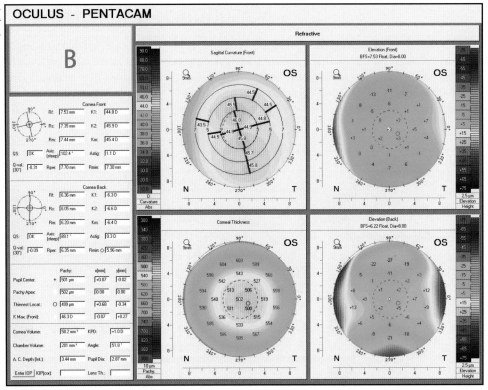

Figure 7-23. This patient's 4-map refractive view shows what appears to be posterior steepening. On slit-lamp examination, the patient was noted to have Salzmann's nodular dystrophy.

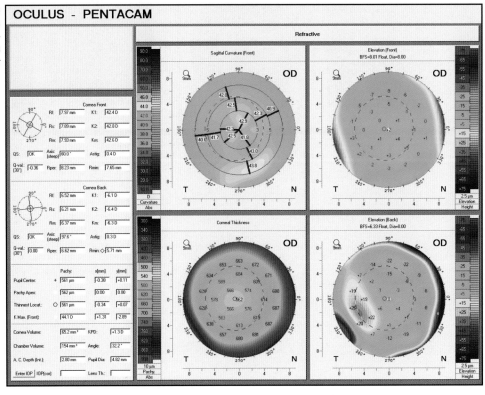

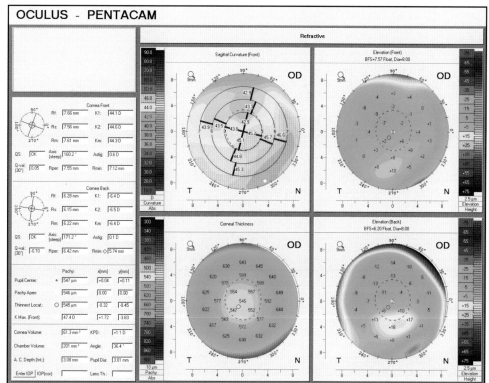

Figure 7-24. This patient's scans show posterior steepening and relative steepening on the sagittal map. However, this is an example of decentered laser-assisted in-situ keratomileusis (LASIK).

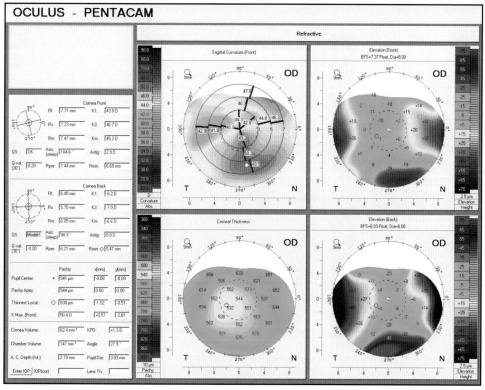

Figure 7-25. If analyzing this topography image without knowledge of the clinical history, one may easily conclude the patient has keratoconus. However, this eye does not have keratoconus, but rather it has Salzmann's nodular degeneration. The Salzmann's is masquerading as keratoconus on the topography image.

Figure 7-26. Slit-lamp photograph of the eye shown in Figure 7-25.

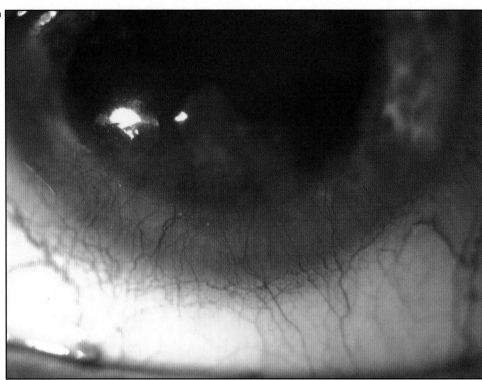

Figure 7-27. Viewing the axial power map alone would suggest that this patient has keratoconus. However, the superior displacement of the thinnest point in the pachymetric map is not consistent with this diagnosis. Clinical examination reveals that the superior thinning is caused by Terrien's marginal degeneration.

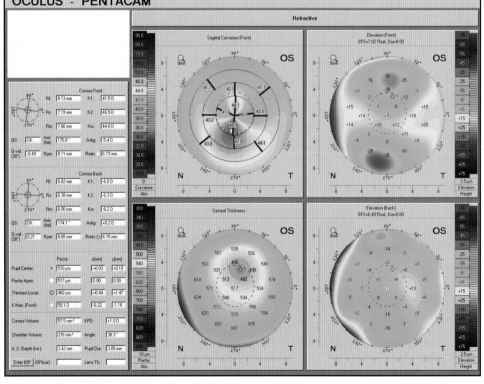

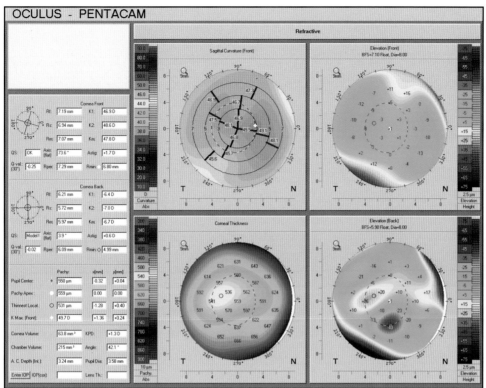

Figure 7-28. Noting the elevation on the posterior surface of this patient's cornea would lead to an initial diagnosis of keratoconus. However, on slit-lamp examination, this patient was diagnosed with posterior polymorphous corneal dystrophy.

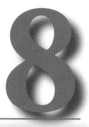

Pellucid Marginal Degeneration

Similar in findings to keratoconus, pellucid marginal degeneration is characterized by inferior peripheral thinning of the cornea due to an idiopathic, noninflammatory condition. Generally thought to be a distinct condition from keratoconus, many experts now consider pellucid marginal degeneration to be the same process as keratoconus but occurring in a different area of the cornea, thus generating a unique topographic appearance.

Although high amounts of against-the-rule astigmatism are usually found, typically there is normal central corneal thickness and an intact central epithelium and, thus, lack of corneal scarring. Corneal topography remains the gold standard for diagnosis. Although the crab-claw appearance may be present in patients' topography maps for both keratoconus and pellucid marginal degeneration, additional elevation maps and locations of corneal thinning can differentiate the 2 degenerations. Pellucid marginal degeneration typically has a 1- to 2-mm wide band, or strip, of thinning that is more peripherally located, whereas keratoconic patients usually have an inferior temporal spot or area of thinning in a cone shape.

Another finding in pellucid marginal degeneration topography is that an area of the vertical axis within the central region of the cornea is noticeably flat. The inferior periphery can have extremely high power contours with thinning. In addition, there is often an area between the limbus and the thinning that is clear, without abnormalities.

Wang M, Kugler LJ. *Atlas and Clinical Reference
Guide for Corneal Topography (pp 69-75).*
© 2014 SLACK Incorporated.

Axial Curvature: Anterior

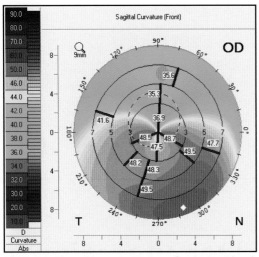

Figure 8-1. The axial curvature maps of patients with pellucid marginal degeneration show marked curvature in the far inferior periphery, as seen in this cornea.

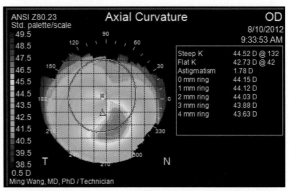

Figure 8-2. Atlas (Carl Zeiss Meditec) topography map of anterior curvature shows an asymmetric crab-claw pattern with inferior steepening.

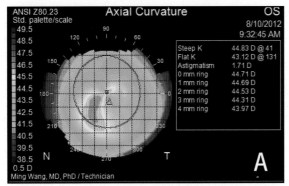

Figure 8-3. (A) Axial curvature with crab-claw appearance, which is typical of pellucid marginal degeneration.

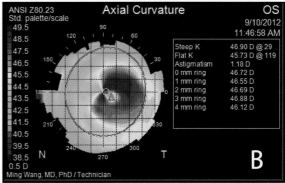

Figure 8-3. (B) The pellucid marginal degeneration crab-claw appearance can present temporally, as seen in this axial curvature map, with an axis of 90 degrees away from typical pellucid marginal degeneration eyes.

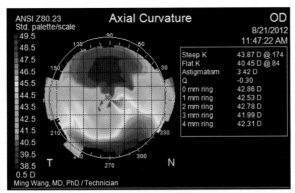

Figure 8-4. Axial curvature map shows the typical pattern of peripheral steepening seen in pellucid marginal degeneration.

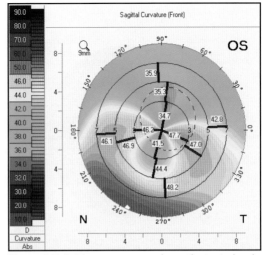

Figure 8-5. Axial curvature map shows the typical crab-claw appearance of inferior cornea in pellucid marginal degeneration.

ANTERIOR ELEVATION

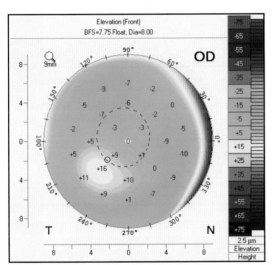

Figure 8-6. Anterior elevation map of a patient with pellucid marginal degeneration shows inferotemporal elevation with a crab-claw appearance of steepening, as seen in the darker green areas.

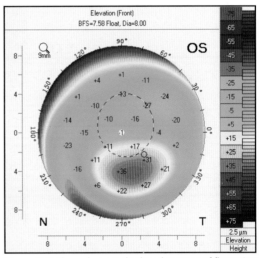

Figure 8-7. Blue colors are displayed as areas of flattening relative to the steeper elevated area inferiorly. This shape produces the crab-claw appearance seen on axial power maps.

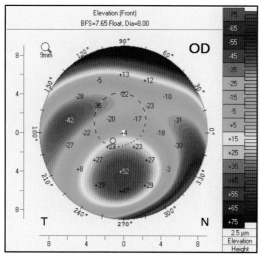

Figure 8-8. This anterior elevation map is an example of inferior elevation, with adjacent flattening, which is typical of pellucid marginal degeneration.

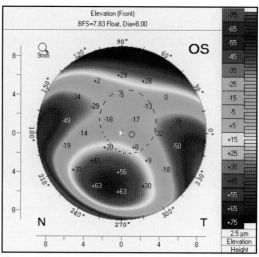

Figure 8-9. Example of severe pellucid marginal degeneration inferiorly, with relative flattening superiorly.

POSTERIOR ELEVATION

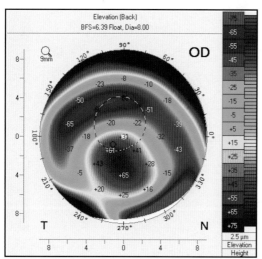

Figure 8-10. As is the case with all corneal ectatic diseases, abnormalities present on the posterior elevation maps before they are detected on the anterior maps. This posterior elevation map shows severe inferior elevation, with relative flattening superiorly.

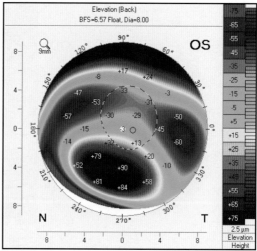

Figure 8-11. A severe case of pellucid marginal degeneration is shown.

PACHYMETRIC MAPS

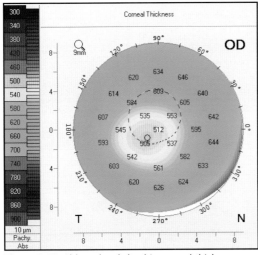

Figure 8-12. Although subtle, this corneal thickness map shows displacement of the thinnest point inferiorly.

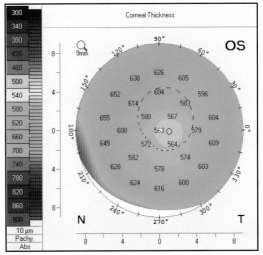

Figure 8-13. Note the oblong asymmetric area of thinning toward the inferotemporal portion of the corneal stroma.

FOUR-MAP REFRACTIVE VIEW

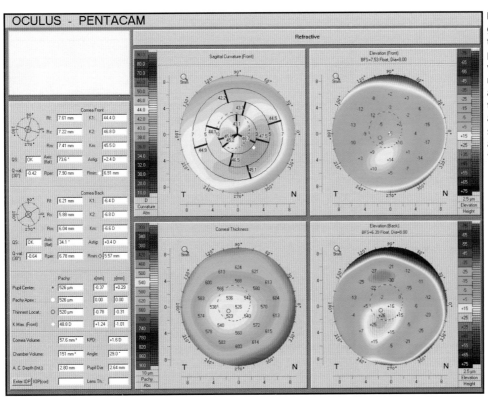

Figure 8-14. As with any topographic study, reviewing all 4 maps together is more beneficial for a proper diagnosis than viewing individual maps. This sagittal curvature map shows a crab-claw appearance. The location of inferonasal thinning is echoed in the anterior and posterior elevation maps, showing irregularities in that same area. The authors call this finding a "3-point touch."

Figure 8-15. This collection of 4 maps is a good illustration of pellucid marginal degeneration, with the classic crab-claw appearance and inferonasal thinning. Pellucid marginal degeneration often has a more elongated area of elevation than the cone shape that is associated with keratoconus.

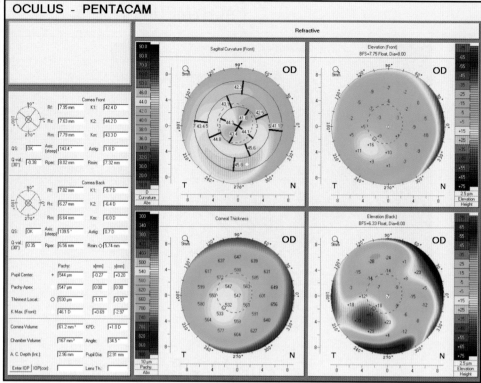

Figure 8-16. This eye, despite having a thicker-than-average cornea, has pellucid marginal degeneration, with severe abnormalities seen in the anterior and posterior elevation maps.

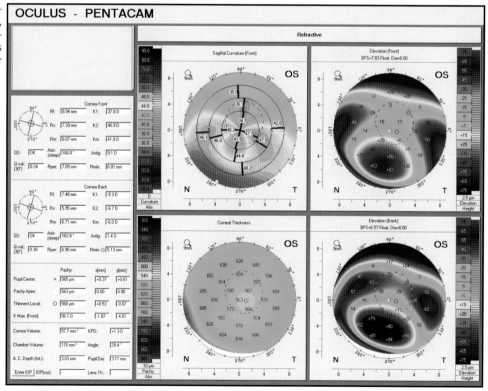

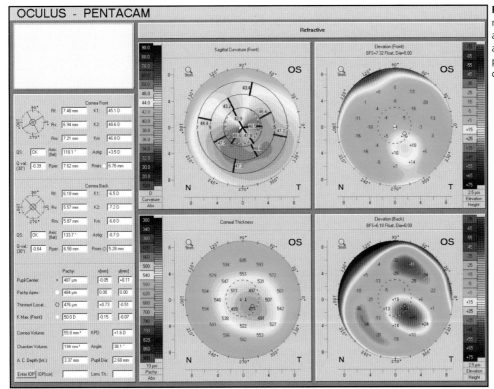

Figure 8-17. Example of pellucid marginal degeneration shows anterior and posterior elevation abnormalities, causing the classic pellucid marginal degeneration changes in anterior curvature.

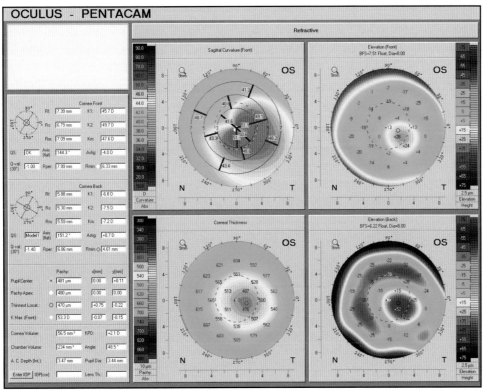

Figure 8-18. Collection of 4 maps illustrates pellucid marginal degeneration with crab-claw pattern steepening in the sagittal curvature map. In addition, the anterior and posterior elevations in the same areas of corneal thinning demonstrate how the cornea is affected. For a definition of pellucid marginal degeneration, these changes should correspond.

Post Refractive Surgery

Post Radial Keratotomy

Eyes with a history of radial keratotomy (RK) have a varied appearance on topography and tomography. Radial keratotomy is inherently an irregular procedure, meaning that the resulting corneal curvature postoperatively is less predictable than with excimer laser surgery. However, RK eyes typically have flat central corneas that are markedly flatter than the periphery. Radial keratotomy incisions often have significant intrastromal scarring and opacity, which causes erroneous interpretation of shape and elevation by imaging devices. Radial keratotomy incisions may also elevate anteriorly, causing focal areas of elevation on topography. Several examples of post-RK eyes are discussed in detail in this section.

Wang M, Kugler LJ. *Atlas and Clinical Reference Guide for Corneal Topography (pp 77-124).*
© 2014 SLACK Incorporated.

Axial Curvature: Anterior

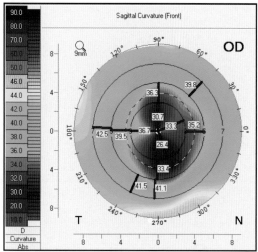

Figure 9-1. Axial curvature map of a patient who had RK surgery. This power map shows keratometry (K) readings from the flat meridian (blue) at 26.40 diopters (D) and in the steep meridian at 42.50 D. Post-RK eyes may often be distinguished from eyes post-excimer laser surgery because of the high degree of irregularity, as well as the severe flattening. It would be unusual to flatten an eye to this degree with an excimer laser.

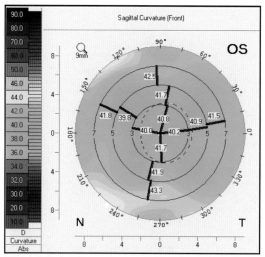

Figure 9-2. Axial curvature map shows irregular astigmatism in a patient who had RK, and the meridians are not 180 degrees apart. In addition, there appears to be noticeable steepening in a butterfly pattern in the darker green areas, which corresponds with the areas of incisions.

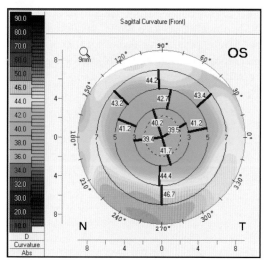

Figure 9-3. Sagittal curvature map shows irregular astigmatism, as well as inferior steepening (orange). A relatively small 5-mm optical zone is noted centrally.

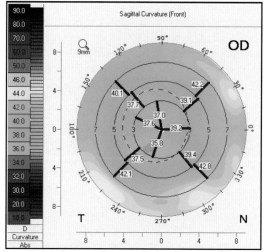

Figure 9-4. Sagittal curvature map of a post-RK patient, with flatter K readings of 35.80 D. A noticeable butterfly pattern is seen, corresponding with the RK incisions.

Anterior Elevation

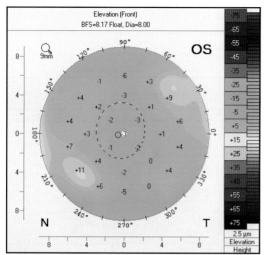

Figure 9-5. This map shows subtle central flattening relative to the peripheral elevation.

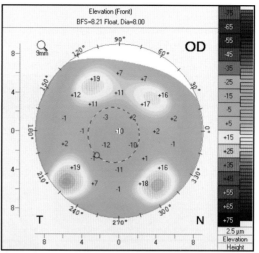

Figure 9-6. Anterior elevation map shows areas of focal increased elevation, corresponding with the RK incisions. The central area of flattening is small and typical of RK optical zones.

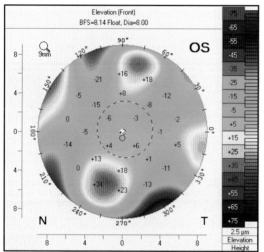

Figure 9-7. Anterior elevation map of a post-RK patient shows 4 distinct areas of elevation (red) associated with the treatment, with relative flattening. The severely elevated areas are suggestive of artifact from RK incisions that have significant scarring or opacity.

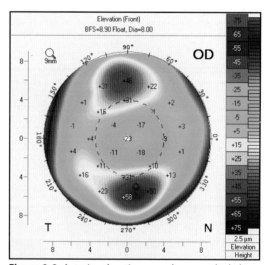

Figure 9-8. Anterior elevation map shows marked elevation in the superior and inferior corneas (red). This appearance is consistent with astigmatic keratotomy incisions at the 90- and 270-degree meridians.

Posterior Elevation

As a general rule, the posterior elevation map does not change significantly after corneal refractive surgery because the refractive procedures exert their effect on the anterior surface. However, RK is the exception to this rule as it works by flattening both the anterior and posterior corneal surfaces.

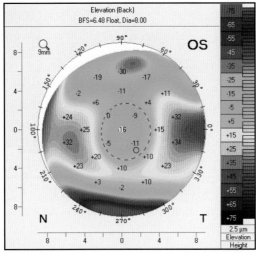

Figure 9-9. The peripheral posterior elevation abnormalities and central flattening shown are consistent with RK.

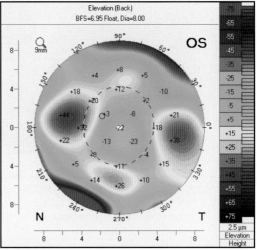

Figure 9-10. Posterior elevation map of a patient who had RK surgery shows marked areas of elevation relative to the incision locations.

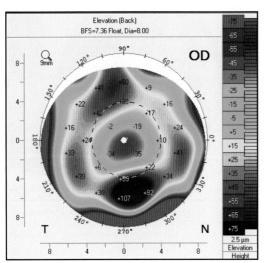

Figure 9-11. The eye shown had a 16-incision RK and now has marked elevation circumferentially in the midperiphery.

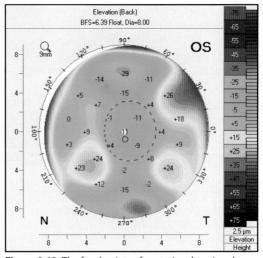

Figure 9-12. The focal points of posterior elevation shown are consistent with a post-RK eye.

Pachymetric Maps

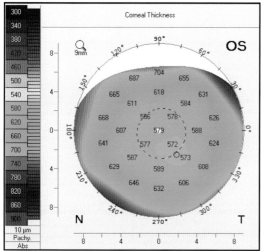

Figure 9-13. Pachymetric map of a post-RK patient shows an irregular contour. However, note the normal central thickness. Because RK does not remove tissue, the central corneal thickness remains normal.

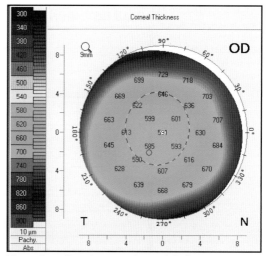

Figure 9-14. Note the normal central thickness.

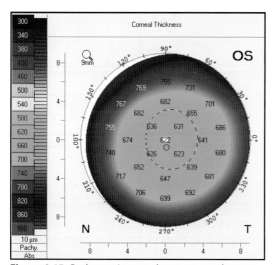

Figure 9-15. Pachymetric map shows a normal progression from center to periphery. There is no way to detect from this pachymetric map that this eye has had prior refractive surgery.

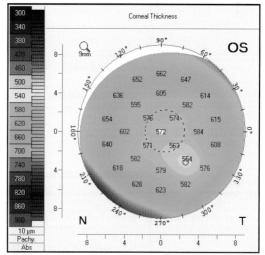

Figure 9-16. Pachymetric map shows an almost cloverleaf appearance of thickness progression, indicating an RK with 4 incisions.

Four-Map Refractive View

Figure 9-17. Central irregularity on axial power and anterior elevation, combined with normal posterior elevation and normal central thickness are classic for RK. This eye had 4 small incisions, hence the mild topographic changes.

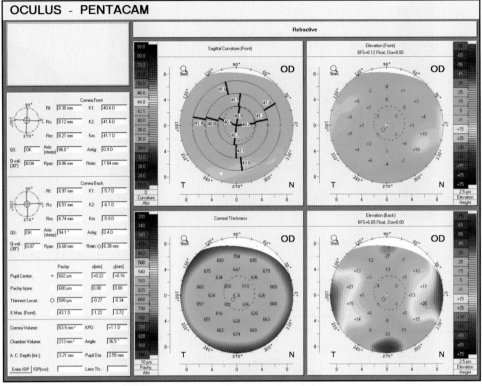

Figure 9-18. Central flattening on this axial power map may be distinguished from LASIK or photorefractive keratectomy (PRK) by the posterior elevation and pachymetric maps. The severe elevation abnormalities on the posterior surface are consistent with RK but would not be present in a post-excimer laser eye. The normal central thickness is also unique to RK.

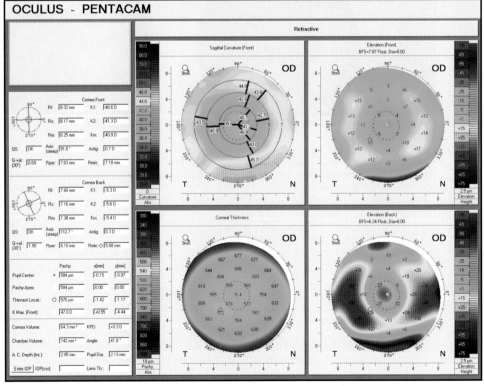

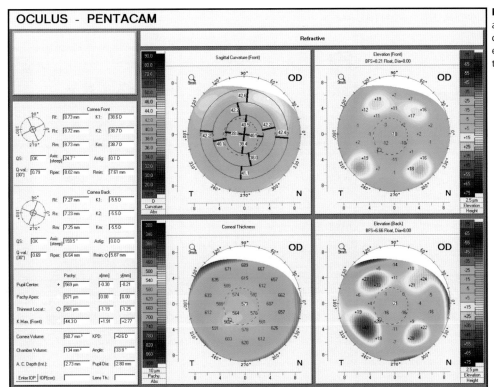

Figure 9-19. Central flattening on axial and anterior maps is from RK due to the focal areas of increased elevation on the anterior and posterior elevation maps.

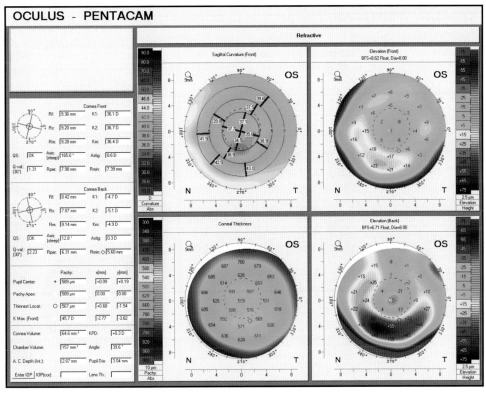

Figure 9-20. Area of increased elevation on the posterior elevation map may be distinguished from post-LASIK ectasia by the areas of focal elevation in the axial power map. The thinnest point on the pachymetric map would be expected to be significantly less than 569 μm if this were an ectatic eye.

Figure 9-21. The focal areas of increased elevation shown are consistent with RK. The irregular curvature on the axial map is also classic.

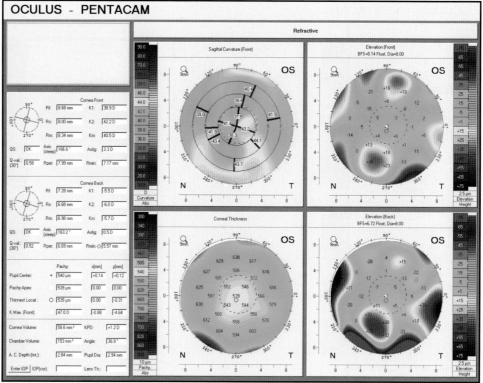

Figure 9-22. The focal areas of increased elevation, combined with central flattening and normal central thickness, are classic for post-RK.

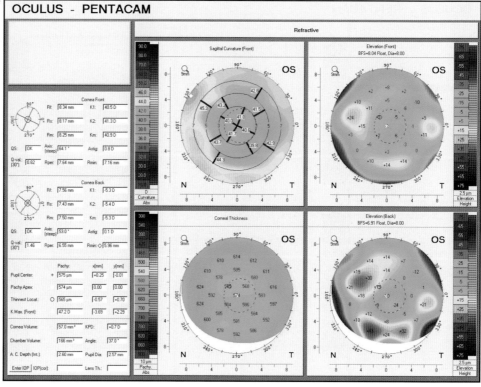

POST PHOTOREFRACTIVE KERATECTOMY

Eyes with a history of prior excimer laser surgery, either PRK or LASIK, have similar appearances. In eyes with prior myopic treatment, there is central flattening relative to the periphery. This results in flatter simulated K readings on the axial power maps. The opposite is true of eyes with prior hyperopic treatment because tissue is removed from the periphery to induce a relative steepening centrally.

Anterior elevation maps are particularly important in eyes with prior excimer laser surgery, as excimer laser procedures remove tissue from the anterior corneal surface.

Axial Curvature: Anterior

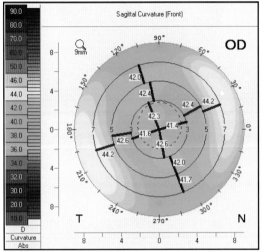

Figure 9-23. Anterior curvature map shows symmetric flattening, which is often seen with post myopic astigmatic PRK patients.

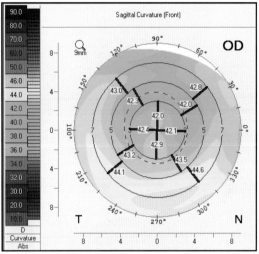

Figure 9-24. The inferior steepening on the axial curvature map is enhanced by the off-center myopic ablation. The steep area may be confused as ectasia, but it is a normal finding that is representative of the step-off from the flat central ablation.

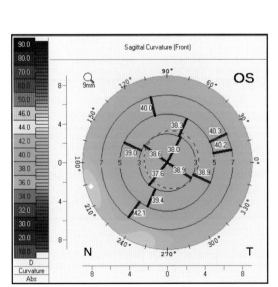

Figure 9-25. Anterior curvature map of a post-PRK patient shows central flattening, which is typical in myopic treatments.

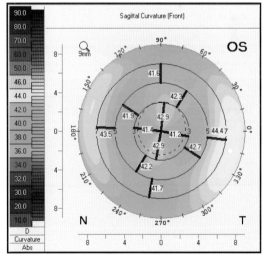

Figure 9-26. Anterior curvature map shows normal postoperative findings for a myopic astigmatic PRK treatment.

Anterior Elevation

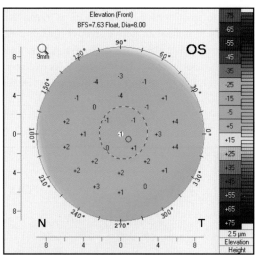

Figure 9-27. Anterior elevation map shows normal findings post-PRK. The mild treatment performed makes this eye difficult to distinguish from a virgin eye.

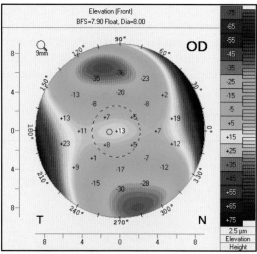

Figure 9-28. Post-PRK anterior elevation map shows an eye after with-the-rule astigmatism treatment. Note that the central 6-mm optical zone is relatively spherical.

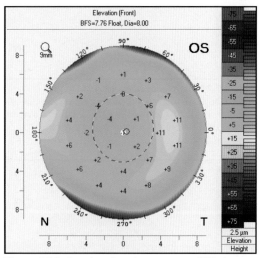

Figure 9-29. Anterior elevation map post-PRK shows a slightly decentered myopic ablation.

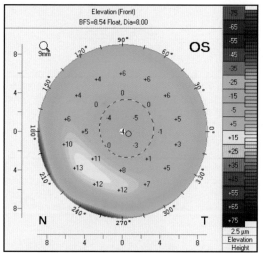

Figure 9-30. Postoperative PRK anterior elevation maps often show uniform flattening in the central 6-mm treatment area, as seen in this map (dark green). Relative steepening (yellow) in the inferotemporal region of the cornea is normal.

Posterior Elevation

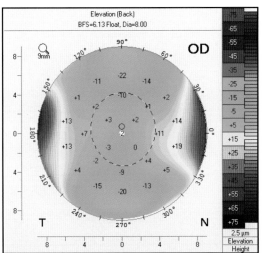

Figure 9-31. Posterior elevations of post-PRK patients should have normal findings, as seen with this map. Excimer lasers remove tissue from the anterior surface but have no effect on the posterior surface.

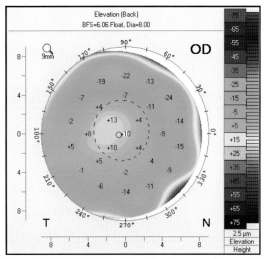

Figure 9-32. Post-PRK posterior elevation map shows mid-peripheral flattening, which is consistent with hyperopic PRK, where the peripheral cornea is treated to create a relatively steeper central area (yellow).

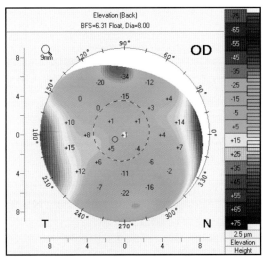

Figure 9-33. Posterior elevation map is consistent with an eye that has significant with-the-rule astigmatism.

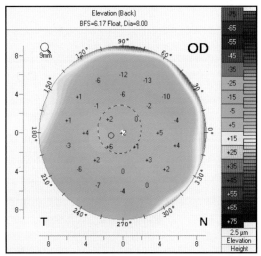

Figure 9-34. Posterior elevation map is normal and demonstrates that the posterior surface is unchanged by excimer laser treatment.

Pachymetric Maps

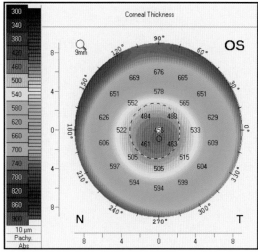

Figure 9-35. Photorefractive keratectomy treatments often result in symmetric distribution on the cornea. This pachymetric map shows uniform thinning in the central cornea (red), with a symmetric increase in thickness to the periphery, which is reflective of the blend zone typical of most modern ablation profiles.

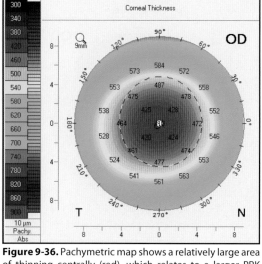

Figure 9-36. Pachymetric map shows a relatively large area of thinning centrally (red), which relates to a larger PRK optical zone with a blend in the periphery.

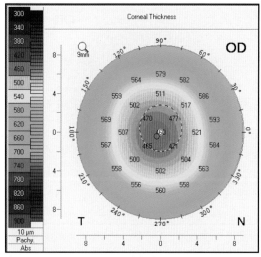

Figure 9-37. Post-PRK corneal thickness map shows normal symmetric thicknesses, with a well-centered ablation zone.

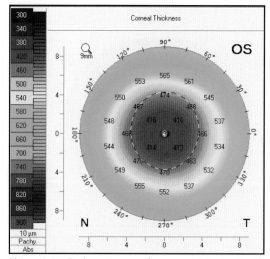

Figure 9-38. Pachymetric map for a post-PRK patient with a normal finding for post myopic treatment.

Four-Map Refractive View

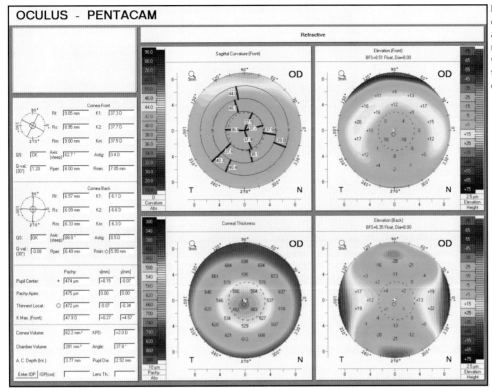

Figure 9-39. The combination of central flattening on axial power and anterior curvature, with normal posterior curvature and a well-centered symmetric area of thinning is classic for post myopic excimer laser treatment.

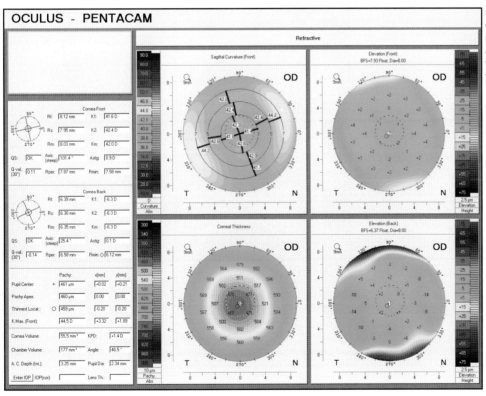

Figure 9-40. The elongated zone of flattening at the 115-degree meridian on the axial power and anterior curvature map is consistent with a post myopic astigmatic treatment.

Figure 9-41. Note that even the large treatment zone with significant corneal thinning does not change the appearance of this posterior corneal elevation map.

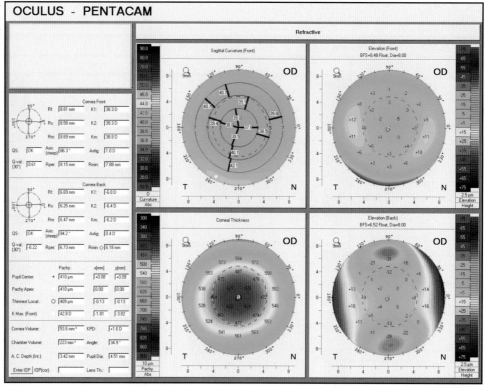

Figure 9-42. A milder myopic ablation is best seen on the anterior elevation map.

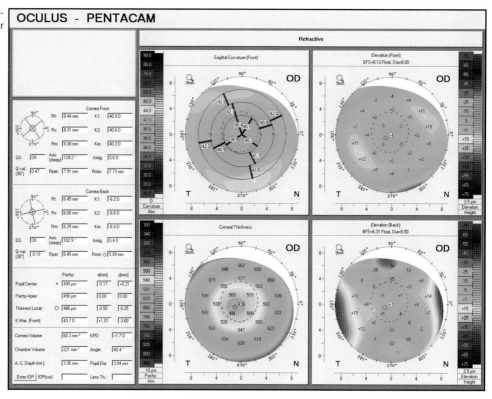

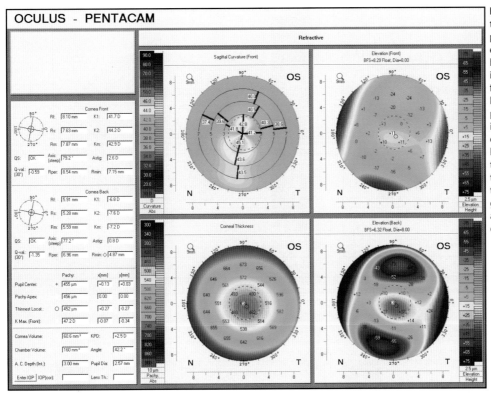

Figure 9-43. It is unusual to see this much astigmatism on the axial power map of an eye after myopic excimer treatment. This eye had a high amount of astigmatism arising from the posterior corneal surface prior to surgery. The excimer laser treatment neutralized the posterior corneal cylinder by imprinting the inverse correction on the anterior corneal surface, hence the abnormal axial astigmatism. Note that the astigmatism on the axial power map is confined to the central 6 mm, which is suggestive that it was imprinted by a laser as opposed to a natural occurrence.

POST-MULTIPLE CORNEAL REFRACTIVE SURGERIES

This section refers to patients who have had more than one refractive surgery procedure. The main point of this section is that the more ablations performed on a given eye, the more chance there is for irregularity.

Axial Curvature: Anterior

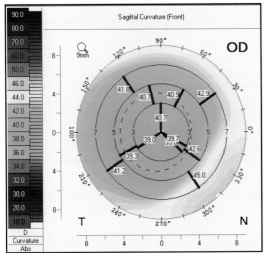

Figure 9-44. Anterior curvature map is post-PRK, plus an enhancement performed several years later. The central visual axis shows normal flattening. Note there is some irregularity centrally.

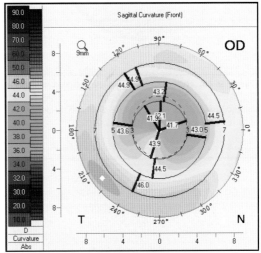

Figure 9-45. This patient had PRK 2 times over the course of several years. Note the small optical zone, which is less than 5 mm.

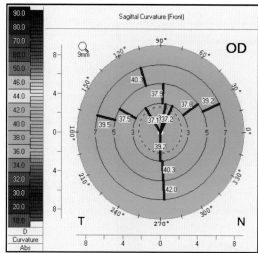

Figure 9-46. Sagittal curvature map shows flattening, which is typically seen in myopic refractive surgery patients. This patient had undergone 2 separate PRK treatments. Irregular astigmatism is seen centrally.

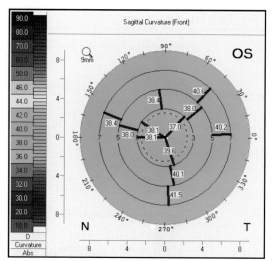

Figure 9-47. Example of irregular astigmatism resulting from multiple excimer procedures.

Anterior Elevation

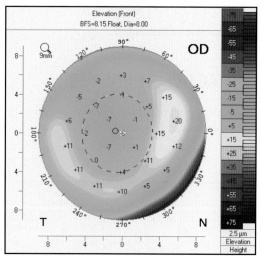

Figure 9-48. This map shows a decentered ablation. It is likely that the decentration led to the need for an enhancement. It is also possible that the decentration occurred as a result of the enhancement.

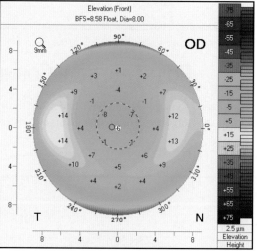

Figure 9-49. This patient had 2 PRK surgeries resulting in central flattening and relative midperipheral elevation. Because the elevation is asymmetrically distributed to the nasal and temporal cornea, it is clear one of the PRK procedures was astigmatic. The central flattening suggests one of the procedures was purely spherical.

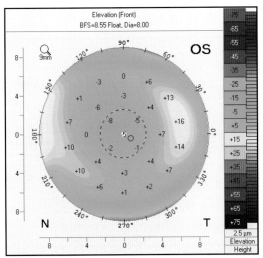

Figure 9-50. Post-PRK anterior elevation map shows normal flattening in the central cornea, with a pattern consistent with myopia and astigmatism

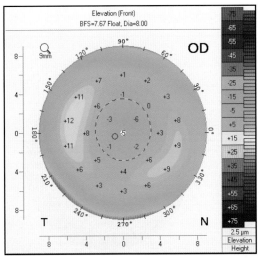

Figure 9-51. Example of a spherical treatment superimposed on an astigmatic treatment.

Posterior Elevation

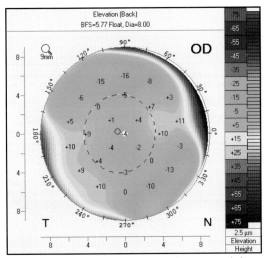

Figure 9-52. Posterior elevation map shows normal elevation after 2 PRK surgeries.

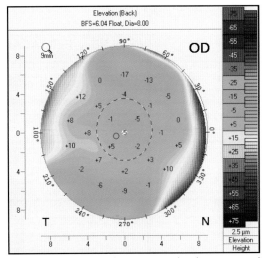

Figure 9-53. Posterior elevation map also shows a normal elevation distribution after multiple PRK surgeries.

Pachymetric Maps

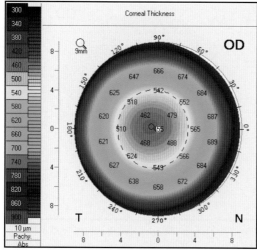

Figure 9-54. Corneal thickness map shows marked drop off from central thinning (red) to midperipheral thicker corneas. This patient had 2 PRK treatments for myopia, both of which removed central corneal tissue.

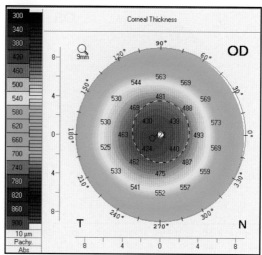

Figure 9-55. The central area of thinning (red) covers an approximate area of 6 to 7 mm, relating to a larger treatment zone with PRK.

Four-Map Refractive View

Figure 9-56. Clinical correlation is required to know with certainty whether this topography is from an eye with multiple surgeries or whether a single surgery induced the findings. However, clearly there is central irregularity on the axial power map and a decentered ablation zone on anterior elevation.

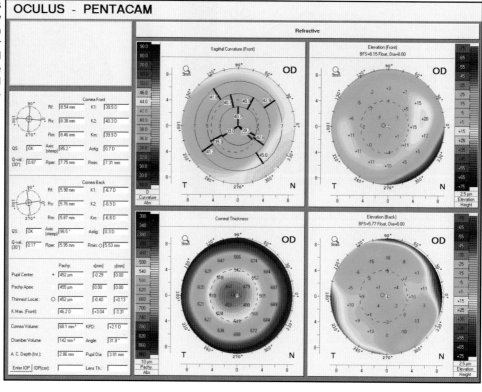

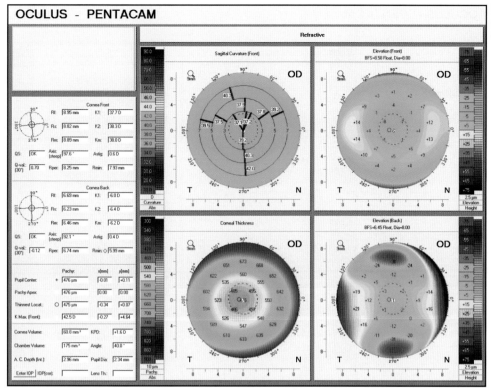

Figure 9-57. Despite multiple surgeries, note the normal posterior elevation map.

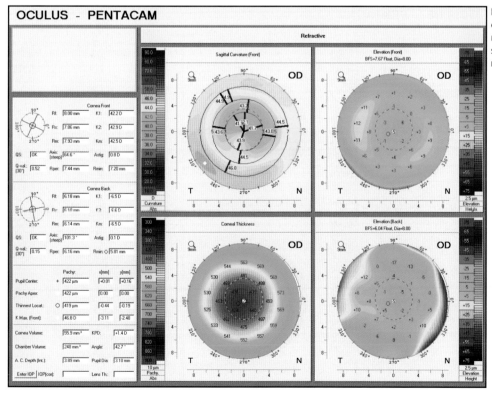

Figure 9-58. The apparent small optical zone on the axial power map and anterior elevation is not significant on the pachymetric map.

Figure 9-59. Note the normal posterior elevation, despite multiple excimer laser surgeries.

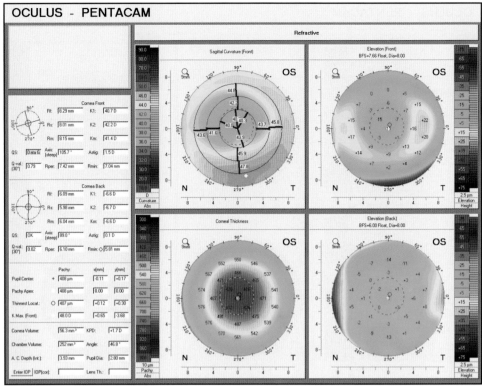

Figure 9-60. Note the central irregularity on the axial power map, with central flattening on anterior curvature and normal posterior curvature.

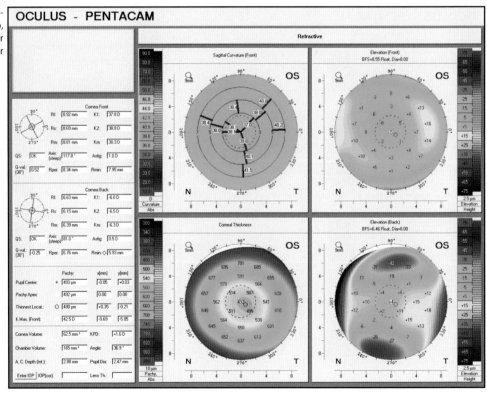

POST-LASIK

Post-LASIK topographies are indistinguishable from post-PRK topographies.

Axial Curvature: Anterior

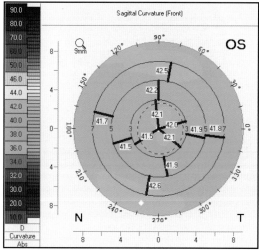

Figure 9-61. Anterior curvature map shows normal curvature, despite prior myopic LASIK.

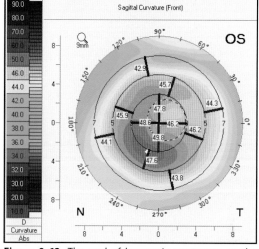

Figure 9-62. The goal of hyperopic treatments on the cornea is to steepen the central area by removing tissue in the midperiphery. This post-LASIK anterior elevation map is typical of a hyperopic treatment, although there is more irregularity centrally than is typically expected.

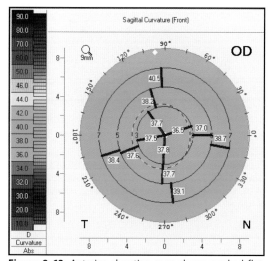

Figure 9-63. Anterior elevation map shows marked flattening centrally due to the high myopic LASIK treatment that was performed.

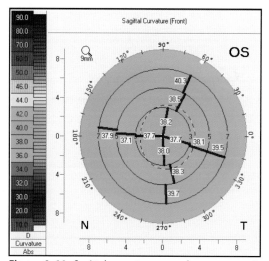

Figure 9-64. Sagittal curvature map shows symmetric flattening across the surface. The patient had a LASIK treatment for high myopia.

Anterior Elevation

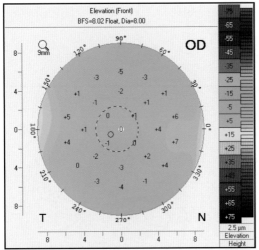

Figure 9-65. Subtle flattening is seen centrally along the 90-degree meridian, which is consistent with myopic astigmatic treatment.

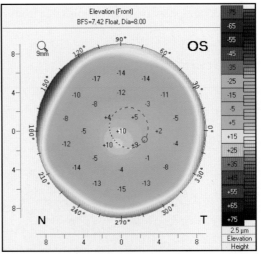

Figure 9-66. Anterior elevation map of a patient treated with hyperopic LASIK. Tissue removal occurred in the midperiphery, resulting in relative elevation centrally. This difference in elevation contributes to steepening and increased refractive power centrally.

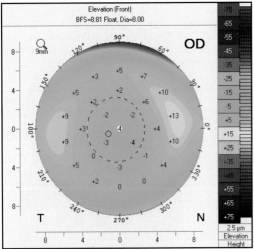

Figure 9-67. High myopic LASIK resulted in this anterior elevation map with central flattening.

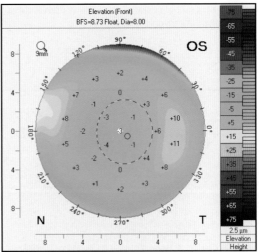

Figure 9-68. This map is an example of post-high myopic LASIK treatment with central flattening, relative to the periphery.

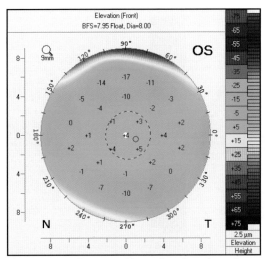

Figure 9-69. Corneas with against-the-rule astigmatism have relative flattening in the periphery of the 180 degree meridian. Excimer laser ablation occurs along the 90 degree meridian in such eyes, resulting in the appearance seen here. Note the flattening along the 180 degree meridian, and areas of decreased elevation superiorly and inferiorly in the 90 degree meridian where the laser energy was applied.

Posterior Elevation

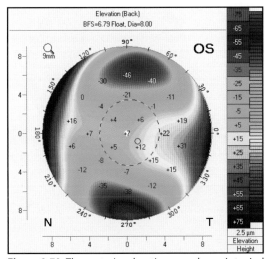

Figure 9-70. The posterior elevation map shown is typical of an eye with high with-the-rule astigmatism.

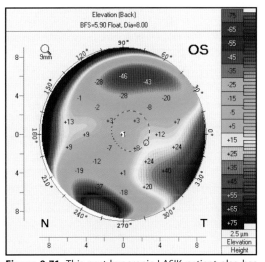

Figure 9-71. This post-hyperopic LASIK patient also has high with-the-rule astigmatism. However, one cannot make that determination from a posterior elevation map.

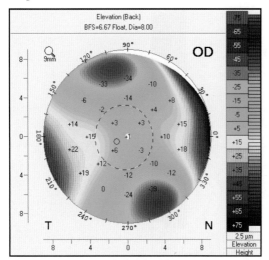

Figure 9-72. Patient with slightly oblique astigmatism, but there is no evidence of treatment in this post-LASIK eye.

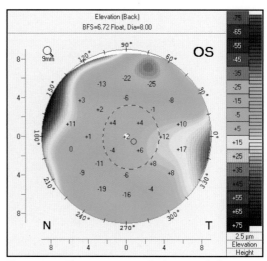

Figure 9-73. This patient was a high myope before LASIK treatment. The posterior elevation map shows no evidence of treatment.

Pachymetric Maps

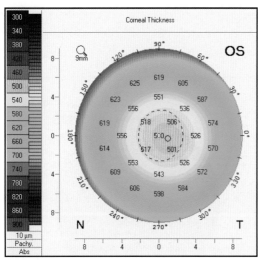

Figure 9-74. Corneal thickness map shows typical postoperative corneal thickness and progression of thickness into the periphery.

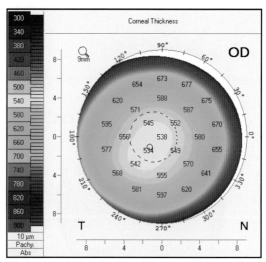

Figure 9-75. This patient had LASIK for hyperopia. Note the circumferential thinning in the periphery relative to the normal center.

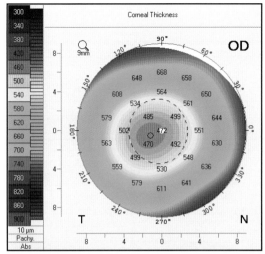

Figure 9-76. Central corneal thickness on this post-myopic LASIK patient is 470 µm, relative to 650 µm in the periphery. Such a large difference would be consistent with keratoconus if this eye had no history of refractive surgery. Another clue that this eye is post surgery rather than having keratoconus is the symmetric and well-centered area of thinning. In a disease state such as keratoconus, the thinnest point would likely be displaced inferiorly.

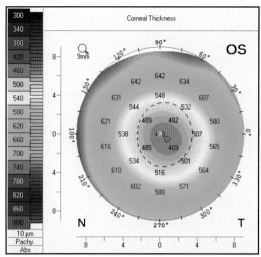

Figure 9-77. Corneal thickness map shows thinnest area of 468 µm after LASIK treatment for high myopia. This is a normal postoperative thickness map for high myopia.

Four-Map Refractive View Preoperative and Postoperatively

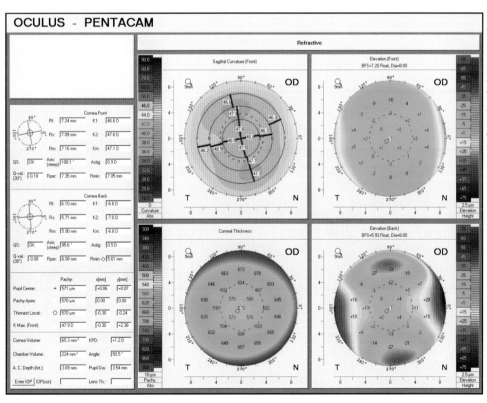

Figure 9-78. This 4-map refractive view shows a patient with a normal cornea. This patient had a relatively high refractive correction prescription, with a mean refractive spherical equivalent of -6.00 D. With a steepest K value of 47.90 D and the thinnest area of the cornea being 570 µm, this patient was a good candidate for LASIK refractive surgery.

Figure 9-79. Postoperative 4-map view for the eye shown in Figure 9-78. The -6.00 D spherical equivalent patient underwent LASIK surgery with this resultant cornea. All 4 maps are normal for post refractive surgery. Note the well-centered ablation and unchanged posterior elevation map.

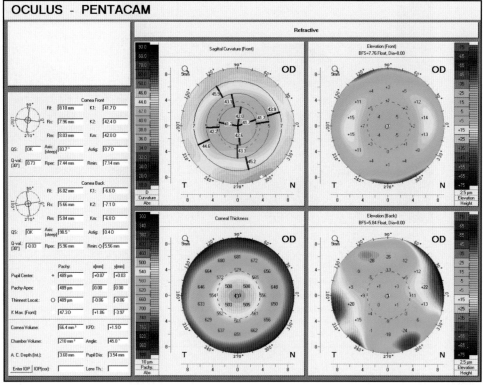

Figure 9-80. This 4-map view represents a low myopic patient with approximately 2.00 D of astigmatism. All parameters are within acceptable ranges for LASIK surgery.

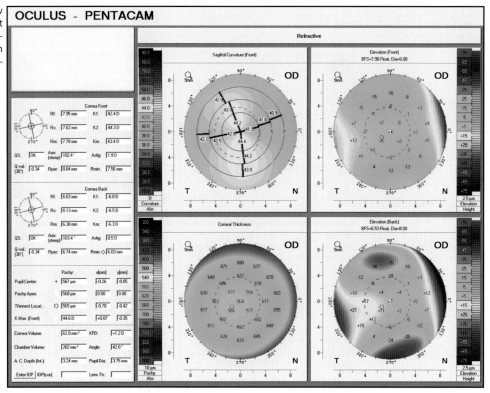

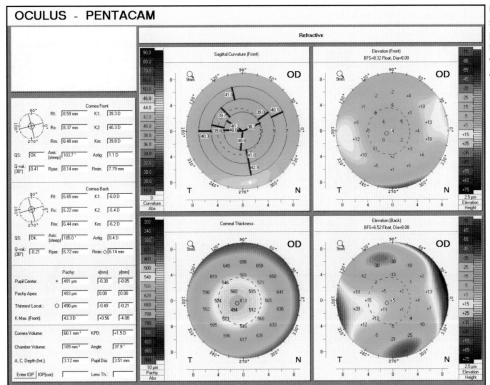

Figure 9-81. This 4-map view shows normal postoperative pictures of the patient shown in Figure 9-80 post-LASIK surgery. All values are within normal ranges for an eye post-LASIK.

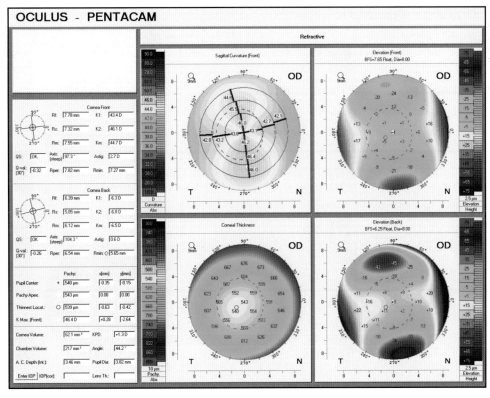

Figure 9-82. These 4 maps show a myopic eye with approximately 3.50 D of astigmatism, as can be seen in the sagittal curvature map. The high astigmatism is mirrored in both the anterior and posterior elevation maps.

Figure 9-83. This 4-map view shows the eye from Figure 9-82 after LASIK surgery. The sagittal curvature map has much less astigmatism, but it has not been completely neutralized.

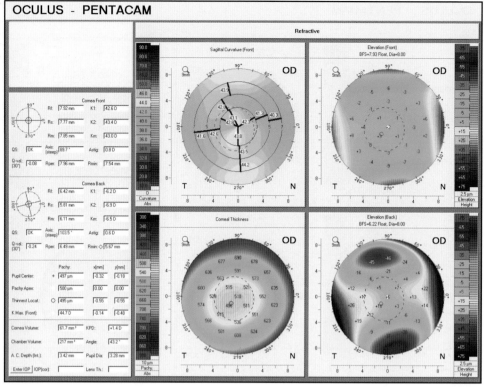

Figure 9-84. Myopic eye with high astigmatism preoperatively.

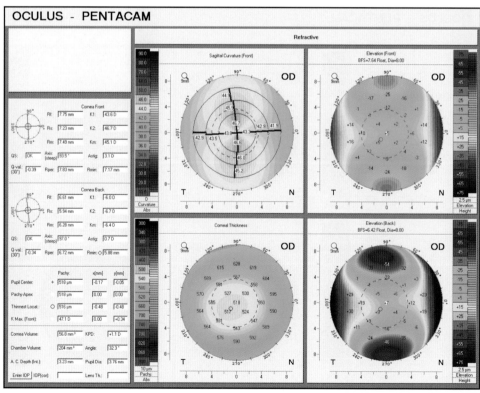

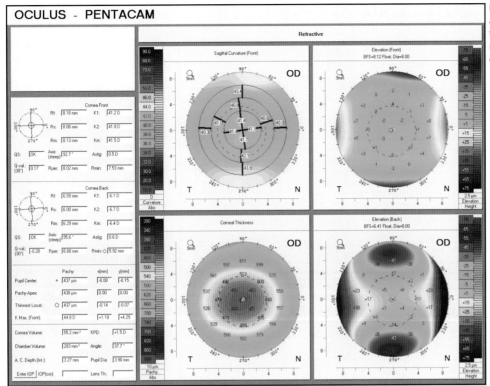

Figure 9-85. Myopic eye with high astigmatism postoperatively. Note the spherical anterior elevation map and the unchanged posterior elevation map.

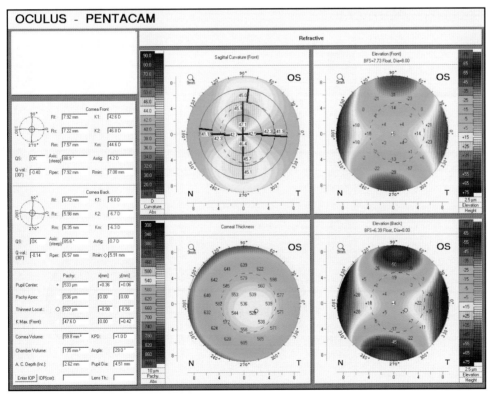

Figure 9-86. Preoperative myopic eye with high astigmatism.

Figure 9-87. Myopic eye with high astigmatism postoperatively. The magnitude of this astigmatism is challenging to completely neutralize.

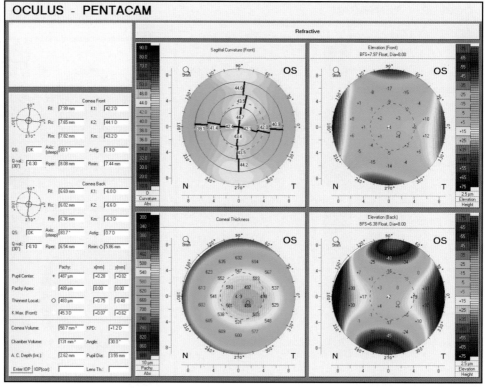

Figure 9-88. Eye with high myopia preoperatively. Although there is inferior steepening on the axial power map, the elevation and pachymetric maps are normal; therefore, there is no diagnosis of subclinical keratoconus. LASIK was subsequently performed.

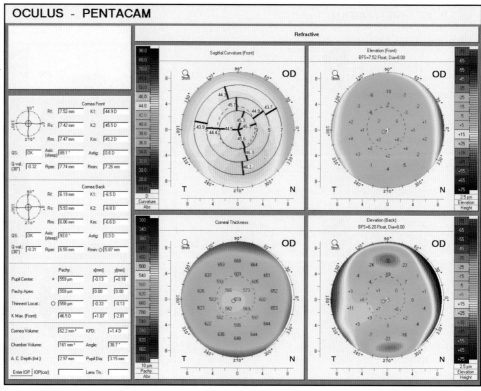

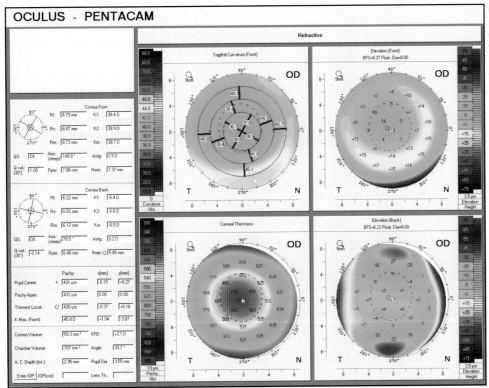

Figure 9-89. Eye with high myopia postoperatively. As clearly seen on the anterior elevation map, the ablation is slightly decentered superiorly. Fortunately, a large ablation zone was used, which is still adequately covering the pupil.

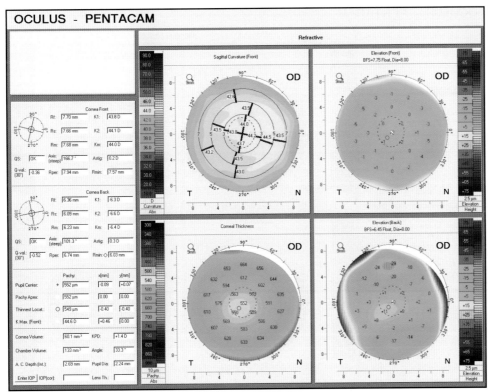

Figure 9-90. Hyperopic eye preoperatively. Although there is a steeper area nasally on the axial power map, there is no corresponding abnormality on the elevation maps.

Figure 9-91. Hyperopic eye 4 months postoperatively. The pattern of peripheral tissue removal is clearly defined on the axial power map and pachymetric map. This change in shape increases the refractive power centrally, as illustrated on the axial power map.

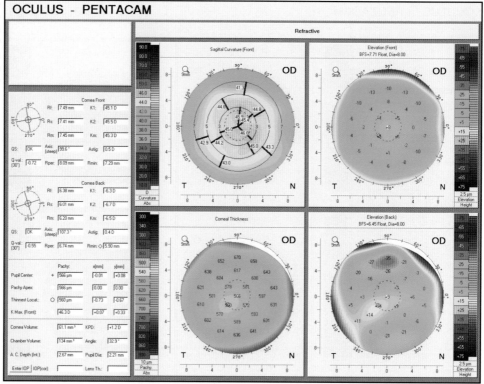

Figure 9-92. High myopia eye with astigmatism preoperatively.

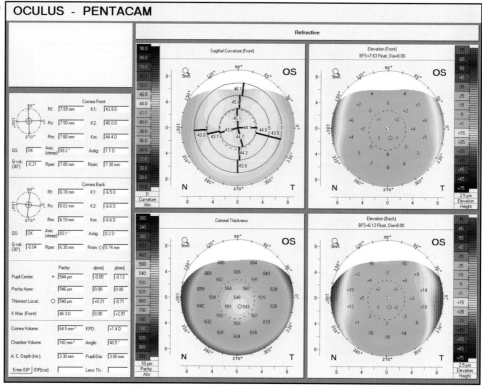

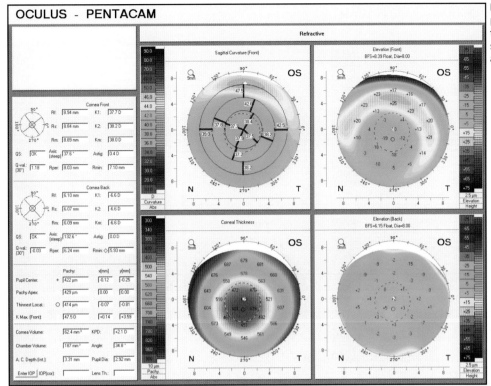

Figure 9-93. High myopia eye postoperatively. This ablation pattern is decentered inferiorly. The step off superiorly is causing the appearance of relative elevation.

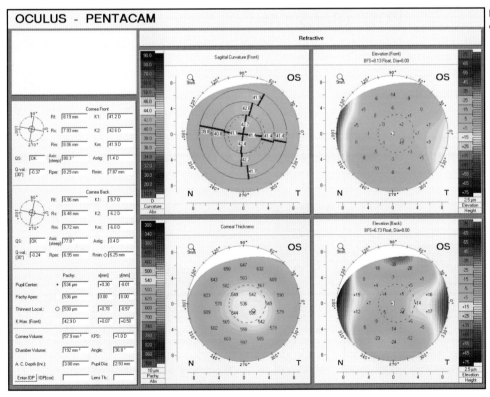

Figure 9-94. High myopia eye preoperatively.

Figure 9-95. High myopia eye postoperatively. An example of a nicely centered myopic ablation.

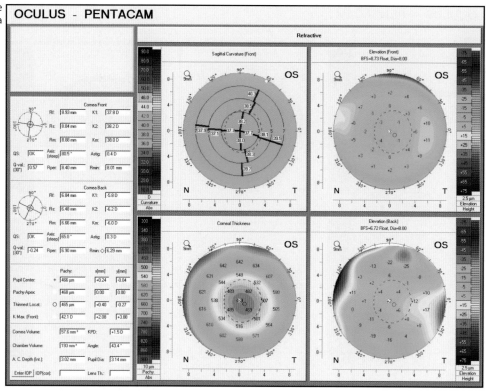

POST TRANSPLANT

Eyes with a history of corneal transplantation have unpredictable and highly variable appearance on topography. In fact, the topographer may interpret the resulting image as an error because the shape varies significantly from any known normal. Several examples of post transplant eyes are described in this section to demonstrate the variety of findings.

Axial Curvature: Anterior

Axial power maps in post penetrating keratoplasty (PKP) eyes typically have high refractive K readings and severe steepening.

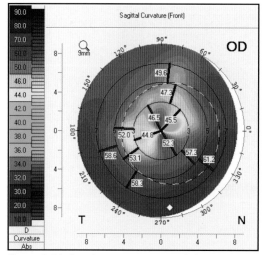

Figure 9-96. Anterior curvature map of this post transplantation patient shows K readings as high as 61.2 D.

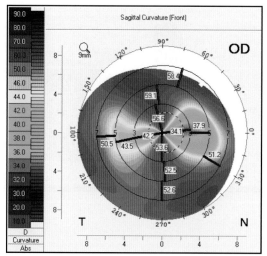

Figure 9-97. Picture of patient who underwent corneal transplant surgery.

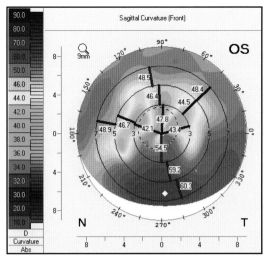

Figure 9-98. Example of a post transplant axial curvature map.

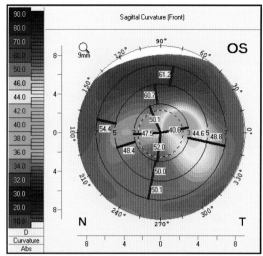

Figure 9-99. Sagittal curvature map shows anterior curvature of 61.20 D.

Anterior Elevation

When describing the surface of a corneal graft relative to a reference sphere, the resulting image may be quite irregular. Almost any pattern is possible.

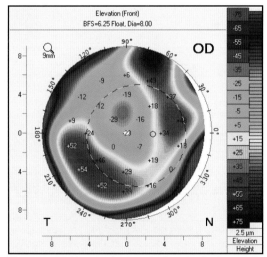

Figure 9-100. Frequently, there is elevation in the periphery at the graft-host junction. This is partly due to the increased elevation in that area and partly due to artifact from peripheral scar tissue.

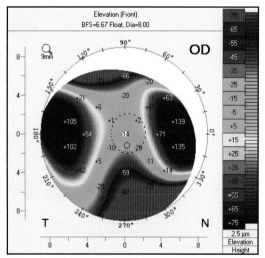

Figure 9-101. Significant peripheral elevation is noted in the nasal and temporal areas of this front elevation map.

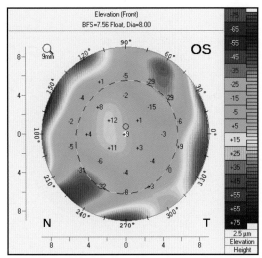

Figure 9-102. Anterior elevation map shows relatively normal findings for a post transplant patient.

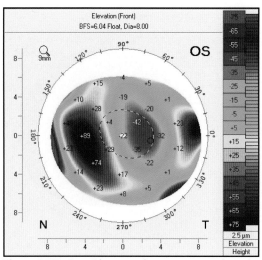

Figure 9-103. Eye with tremendous asymmetry along the 180-degree meridian.

Posterior Elevation

Posterior elevation maps in post-PKP eyes are even more irregular than the anterior elevation maps. The reason is partly because of the difficulty in accurately measuring the posterior surface through an edematous and thick graft.

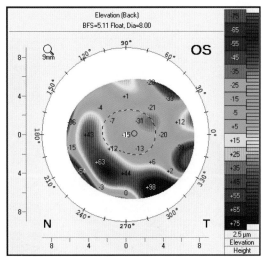

Figure 9-104. Although this is an irregular posterior surface, the high posterior elevation could be due to the fact that most PKP eyes are keratoconic and will have steep posterior surfaces.

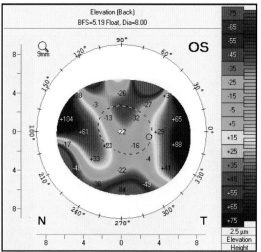

Figure 9-105. Posterior elevation map shows peripheral elevation, most likely due to the irregular surface and difficulty mapping through the transplant.

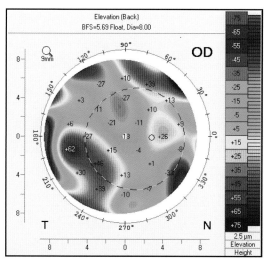

Figure 9-106. Example of a post transplant eye that is irregular, which is expected with the Pentacam (OCULUS Optikgeräte GmbH) after such a surgery.

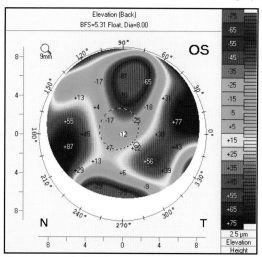

Figure 9-107. This highly irregular posterior elevation map is most likely due to the irregularity of the transplant.

Pachymetric Maps

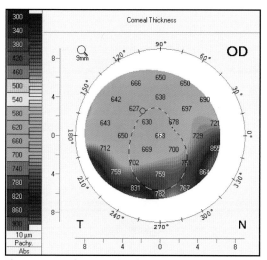

Figure 9-108. This severely edematous graft is failing.

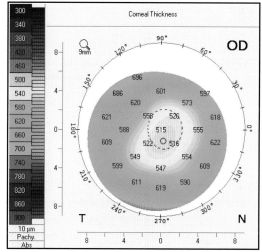

Figure 9-109. Some mild irregularity in the pachymetric distribution is seen, but overall it is normal and is impossible to detect a history of transplantation.

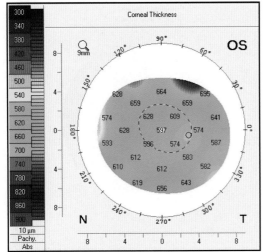

Figure 9-110. The irregular pattern shown is consistent with either early graft failure or artifact.

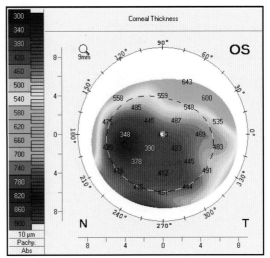

Figure 9-111. Recurrent keratoconus in a graft post transplantation.

Four-Map Refractive View

Figure 9-112. Almost any topographic pattern is possible in eyes after PKP. Note the severe steepening and irregularity.

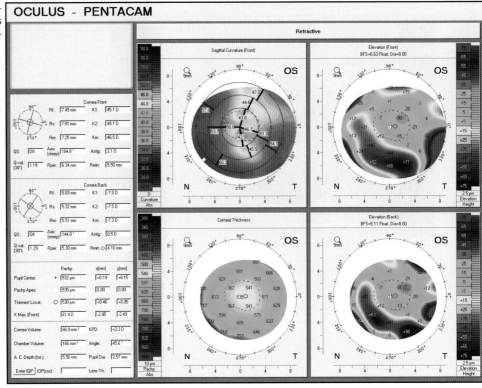

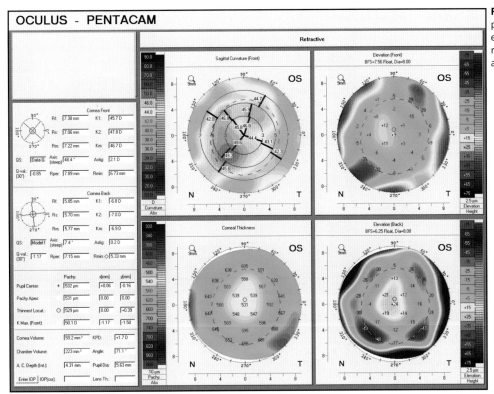

Figure 9-113. Graft that is well positioned and symmetric. This eye could potentially have laser refractive surgery to correct the astigmatism in the graft.

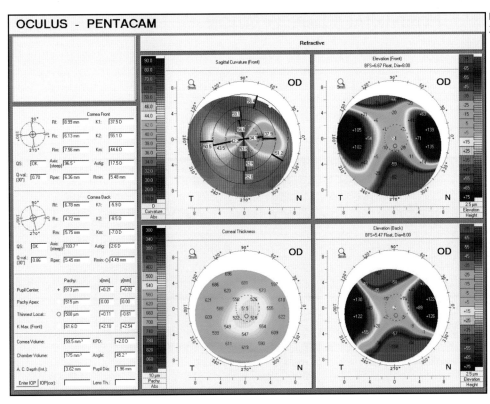

Figure 9-114. Note there is almost 20.00 D of astigmatism in this eye.

Figure 9-115. Eye with high astigmatism, irregularity, and thinning.

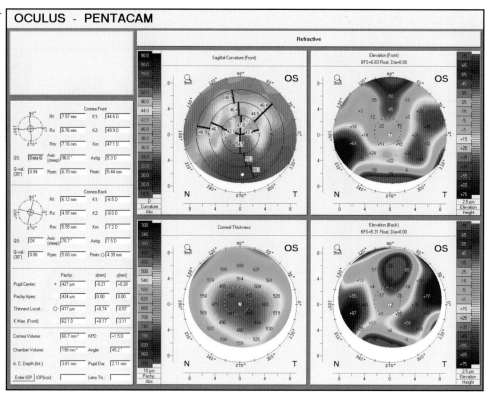

POST-INTACS IMPLANTATION

Eyes with a history of implantation of intrastromal corneal ring segments, such as Intacs, have a characteristic appearance of flattening in the area of the ring implant, with relative steepening in the center. Complicating the topographic appearance of these eyes is the fact that corneal rings are usually implanted in eyes with severe keratoconus.

Axial Curvature: Anterior

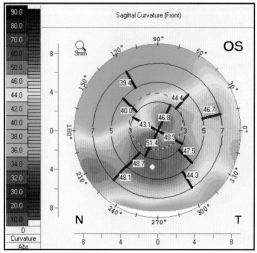

Figure 9-116. The green areas superior and posterior to the central steepening correspond with the Intacs (Addition Technology, Inc) ring segments.

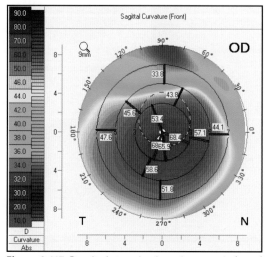

Figure 9-117. Despite Intacs ring insertion superiorly and inferiorly, there is no evidence of flattening in this cornea.

Anterior Elevation

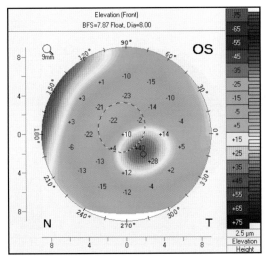

Figure 9-118. The blue areas circumferential to the tip of the cone correspond to the Intacs ring segments.

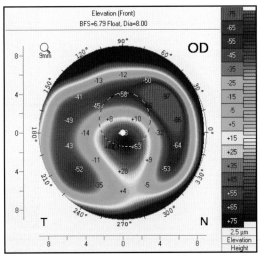

Figure 9-119. Eye with a severe case of keratoconus that had successful Intacs treatment. Note the remarkable difference in elevation between the central apex and the periphery.

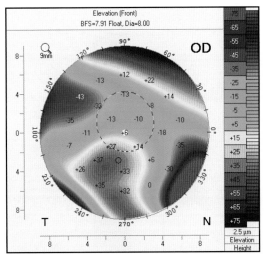

Figure 9-120. This cone is severe to the point where the inferior ring segment only moderately flattened the steep area.

Posterior Elevation

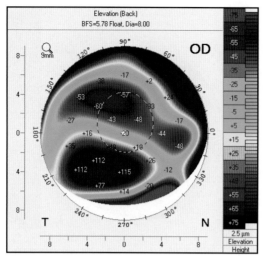

Figure 9-121. Eye with severe keratoconus. The Intacs ring segments are somewhat effective in decreasing the size of the ectatic area.

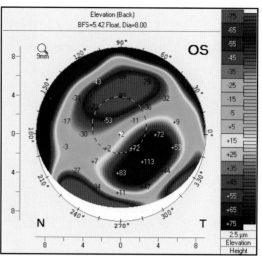

Figure 9-122. Posterior elevation map shows marked changes relating to keratoconus. This patient is post-Intacs implantation.

Pachymetric Maps

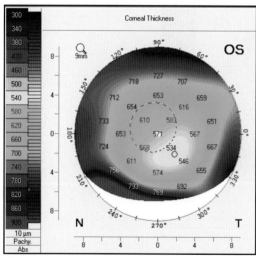

Figure 9-123. Pachymetry map shows a patient post-Intacs implantation. Because the implantation minimally affects the thickness of the cornea, no significant changes to the corneal thickness are noted.

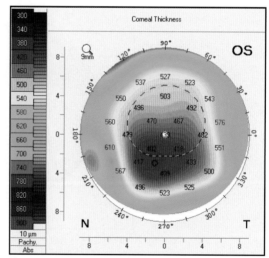

Figure 9-124. Corneal thickness map shows irregular distribution of tissue, which may be due to the preoperative condition the Intacs was treating. Intacs should not affect the overall thickness of the cornea.

Four-Map Refractive View

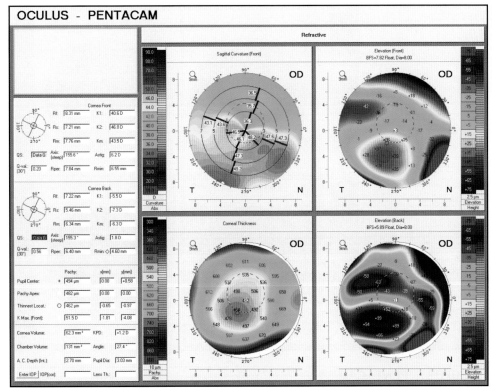

Figure 9-125. Post-Intacs eyes can be difficult to determine on topography alone without knowing the clinical history. However, as is seen in this eye, there is subtle flattening inferiorly in what otherwise would be steeper than the midperiphery.

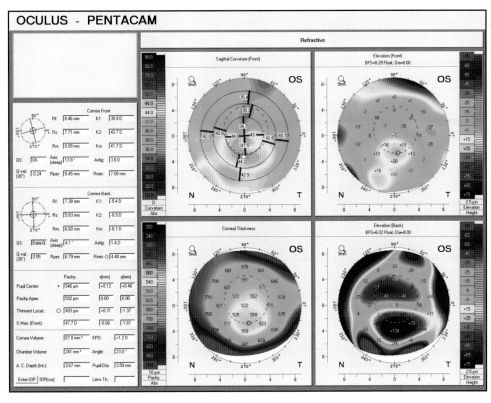

Figure 9-126. The flat zone in the far inferior periphery is the hallmark of topography in post-Intacs eyes.

Figure 9-127. The elevated area inferiorly has been displaced toward the center, opposite of the flattening induced by the Intacs segment.

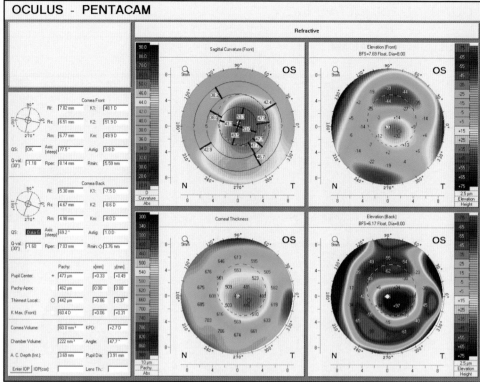

Figure 9-128. Note the flattening in the far inferior periphery.

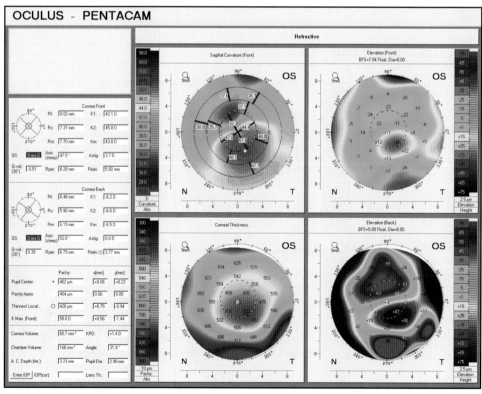

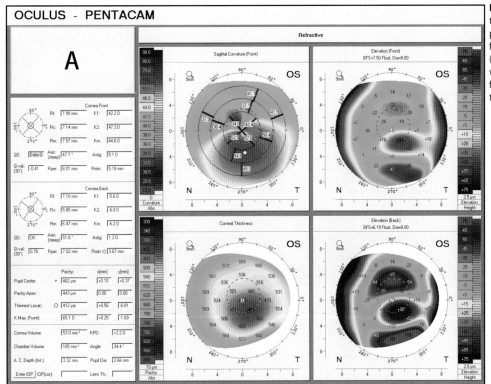

Figure 9-129. (A) Two sets of refractive maps shows a patient pre- and postoperative Intacs implantation for the treatment of keratoconus. (A) Note the posterior elevation, which is mirrored on the front surface and the inferior steepening on the sagittal curvature map.

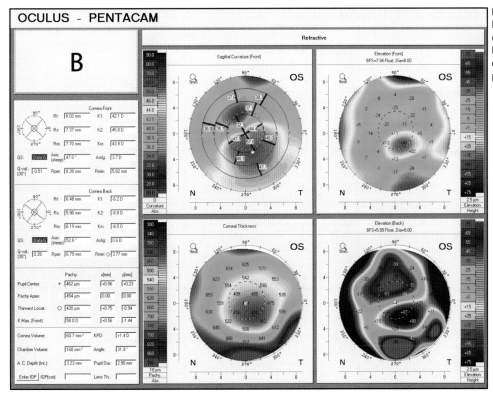

Figure 9-129. (B) Pictures shows how the Intacs decreased the area of the cone on the sagittal surface. Posterior elevation does not always change significantly with Intacs placement.

Figure 9-130. (A) A patient with advanced keratoconus, as can be seen from posterior elevation and steepening on the sagittal curvature map. In addition, the thickness profile shows inferior temporal thinning, which is characteristic of keratoconus.

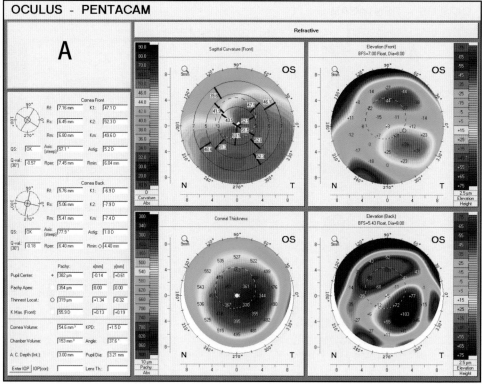

Figure 9-130. (B) Postoperative maps for Intacs. Significant improvement is seen on the sagittal curvature map.

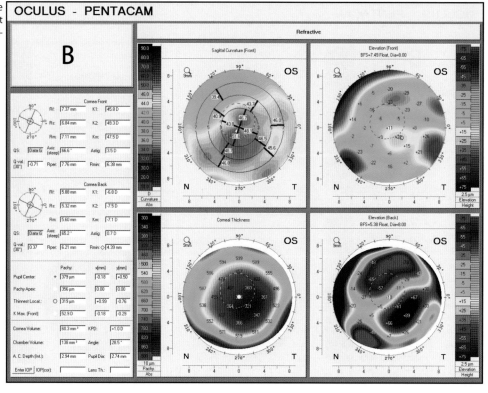

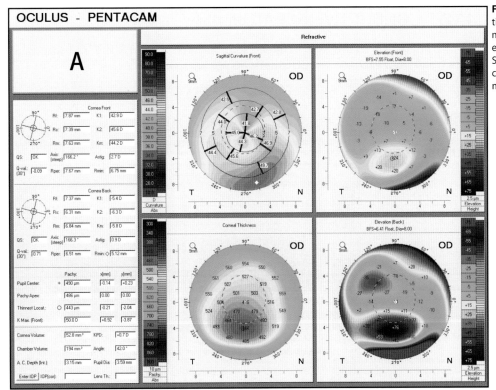

Figure 9-131. (A) Four-map refractive view of a patient with pellucid marginal degeneration. Posterior elevation shows marked elevation. Sagittal curvature map shows the crab-claw appearance of pellucid marginal degeneration.

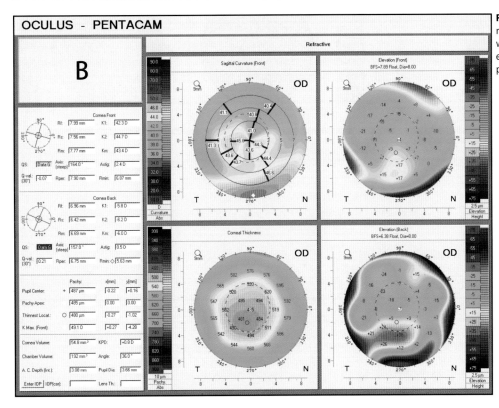

Figure 9-131. (B) Post-Intacs set of refractive pictures for this patient, which shows a marked decrease in elevation in the area of the Intacs placement.

POST CONDUCTIVE KERATOPLASTY

Eyes with a history of conductive keratoplasty (CK) are similar in appearance to eyes with a history of hyperopic LASIK. The stromal scars in CK eyes, however, may cause an irregular appearance in the periphery and may cause artifact in the image interpretation.

Four-Map Refractive View

Figure 9-132. This eye is post-CK, and the findings are very subtle. The K readings centrally are steeper on average, and there is mild flattening circumferentially in the periphery seen best on the anterior elevation map.

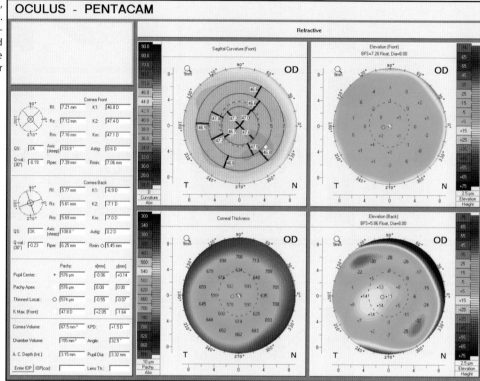

10

Irregular Astigmatism

Irregular astigmatism, by definition, refers to when the principal meridians of the cornea are not oriented 90 degrees apart, and it is often associated with a loss of best-corrected visual acuity. It can also be defined as when different parts of the same meridian have different degrees of curvature from one point to another. When irregular astigmatism has a defined pattern, typically with a steep or flat area of at least 2 mm in diameter, it is classified as macro-irregular astigmatism. Conversely, when there is an indistinct pattern, with multiple irregularities on the cornea, it is defined as micro-irregular astigmatism. With an undefined pattern of astigmatism, the profile maps are difficult to calculate.

This can be due to the presence of corneal dystrophies, such as anterior basement membrane dystrophy; degenerations, such as keratoconus; or post surgical conditions, such as decentered ablations or ectasia. With decentered ablations, topography can improve over time as the epithelium fills in. However, with keratoconus or ectasia, the conditions typically worsen.

Wang M, Kugler LJ. *Atlas and Clinical Reference Guide for Corneal Topography (pp 125-132).*
© 2014 SLACK Incorporated.

AXIAL CURVATURE: ANTERIOR

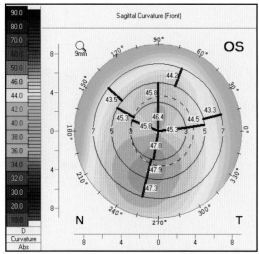

Figure 10-1. The difference between inferior and superior curvature, called the I-S difference, is a common type of irregular astigmatism.

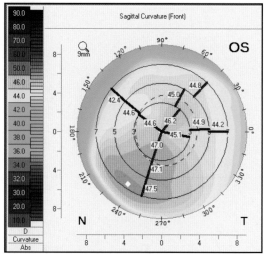

Figure 10-2. Irregular astigmatism is often present in asymmetric corneal curvature, as seen in this anterior curvature map. Steepness in the inferior nasal area offsets the relative flattening in the superior temporal area.

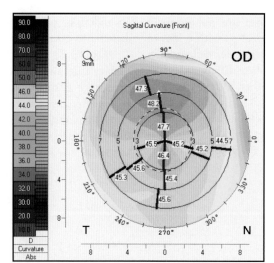

Figure 10-3. The 180-degree meridian shows asymmetric distribution of the curvature across the cornea due to the asymmetric steepening seen in the superior cornea of 48.20 diopters (D).

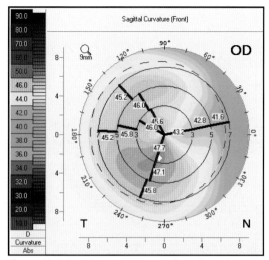

Figure 10-4. Anterior curvature map shows irregular astigmatism with significant asymmetric bow-tie appearance with inferior-temporal steepening.

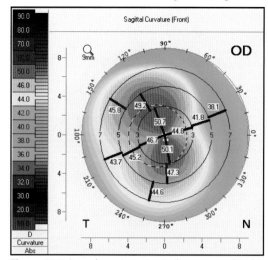

Figure 10-5. Irregular astigmatism is demonstrated in this axial curvature map by changes in the power across multiple points on the cornea.

ANTERIOR ELEVATION

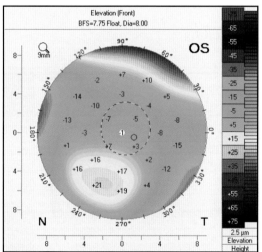

Figure 10-6. The anterior elevation map of this patient's cornea shows inferior nasal elevation and an asymmetric distribution of elevation in comparison with a known sphere, thus causing an irregular corneal shape and irregular astigmatism.

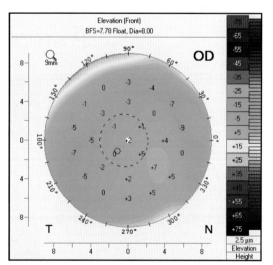

Figure 10-7. Anterior elevation map shows slight irregularity in the surface, although it is difficult to diagnose irregular astigmatism without looking at the anterior curvature map as well.

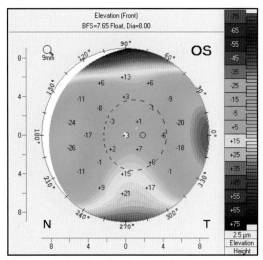

Figure 10-8. Anterior elevation map shows a cornea treated for hyperopic with-the-rule astigmatism by removing tissue in the periphery of the 180-degree meridian, thereby steepening along that meridian centrally. Although the elevation map looks grossly normal, there is a narrower band of elevation superiorly in the optical zone compared with the interior optical zone.

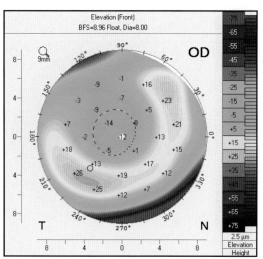

Figure 10-9. Anterior elevation map shows a post myopic refractive surgery cornea. The decentered ablation is causing an irregular corneal shape and inducing irregular astigmatism.

POSTERIOR ELEVATION

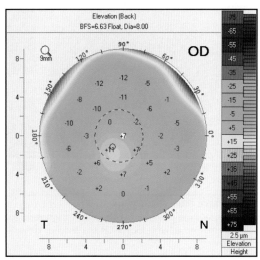

Figure 10-10. Posterior elevation maps can show irregularities prior to anterior surface anomalies. This eye has an area of elevation inferiorly, which may represent early ectatic disease. The irregular shape induces irregular astigmatism in this eye.

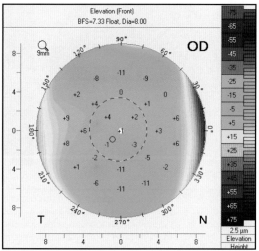

Figure 10-11. Example of a posterior elevation map that appears normal, but the patient has been diagnosed with irregular astigmatism. Observing the posterior elevation map alone typically does not allow the clinician to diagnose a patient with irregular astigmatism.

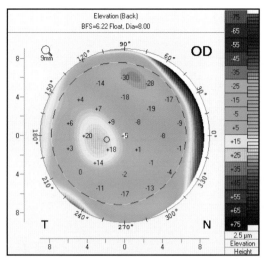

Figure 10-12. Posterior elevation map shows significant elevation in the temporal portion of the posterior cornea. A patient with this finding may have anterior elevation changes as well, leading to a diagnosis of an abnormal cornea. This patient was diagnosed with irregular astigmatism, which was induced by the asymmetric posterior corneal surface.

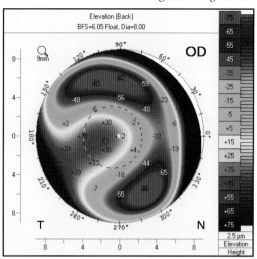

Figure 10-13. If the anterior curvature and elevation maps of this patient were observed, they would most likely mirror some of the abnormalities seen in this posterior elevation map. Obvious posterior elevation in this patient's cornea is seen (red), which is being diagnosed as irregular astigmatism.

PACHYMETRIC MAPS

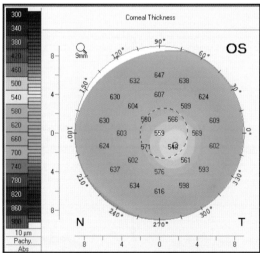

Figure 10-14. Corneal thickness distribution should be thinnest in the central 5 mm, and it should increase uniformly into the periphery, as seen in this pachymetric map. Although the patient was diagnosed as irregular astigmatism, this cornea's pachymetric map appears normal.

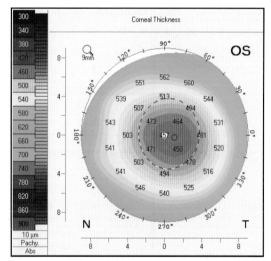

Figure 10-15. Corneal thickness map shows central thinning with some peripheral irregularities that can be associated with post refractive surgical corneas. This patient was diagnosed with irregular astigmatism, although the diagnosis is difficult to make from this pachymetric map alone.

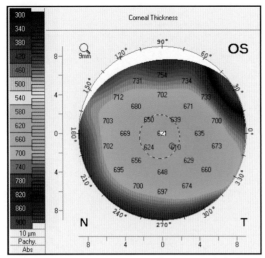

Figure 10-16. Pachymetry map shows central thickness higher than average, with some peripheral distortions. This appearance is consistent with corneal edema, which is inducing the irregular astigmatism seen in the axial power map of this Fuchs' dystrophy patient.

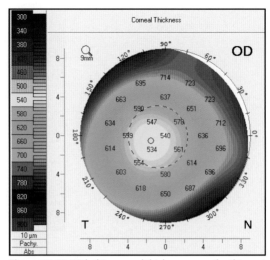

Figure 10-17. With this corneal thickness map, the thinnest area of the cornea is within normal limits. Slight inferotemporal distribution of the thickness distribution could be normal. However, with additional corneal evaluation, this patient was diagnosed with irregular astigmatism.

FOUR-MAP REFRACTIVE VIEW

Figure 10-18. Eye with pellucid marginal degeneration demonstrates how abnormal corneal shape can induce irregular astigmatism, which is best seen on the axial power map.

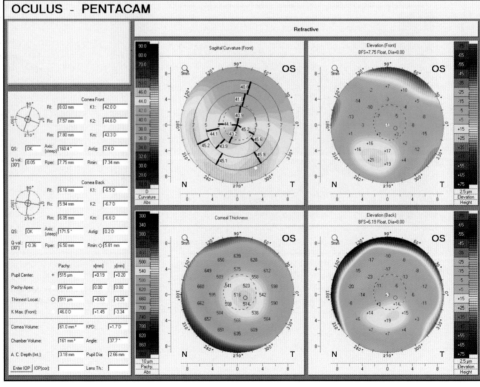

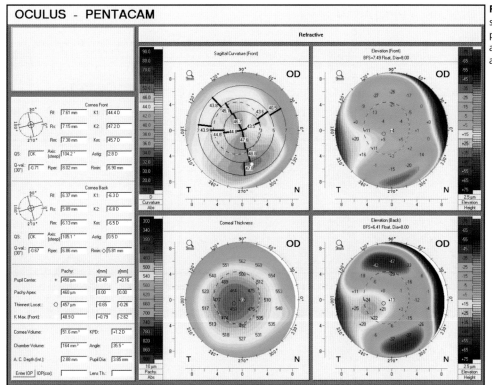

Figure 10-19. Although there is significant irregularity in this axial power map that is causing irregular astigmatism, the elevation maps are grossly normal.

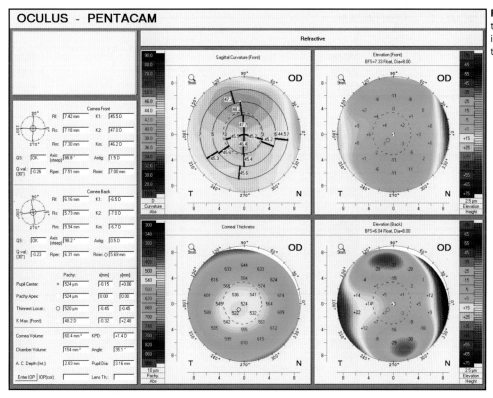

Figure 10-20. Mild asymmetry in the anterior elevation map may be inducing the irregularity seen in the anterior corneal surface power.

Figure 10-21. Sagittal curvature map of this group of refractive maps shows an unusual bent bow-tie appearance in the 90-degree meridian, which is one of the most common types of irregular astigmatism.

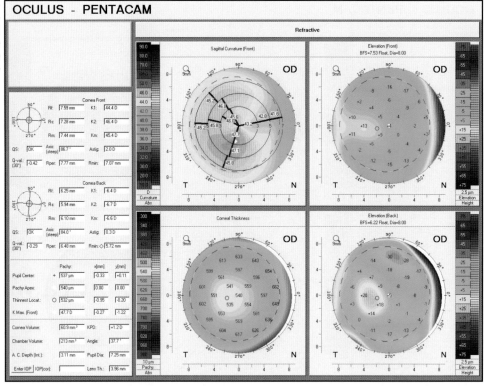

Figure 10-22. Group of maps shows mild bent bow-tie appearance in the 180-degree meridian of the axial power map. The mild irregularity in the anterior and posterior elevation maps describe the shape that leads to the irregular bent bow-tie appearance.

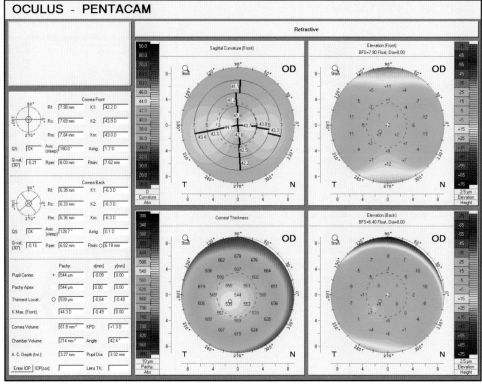

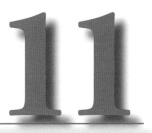

Post Surgical Ectasia

Ectasia is described as progressive thinning and steepening of the cornea, resulting in irregular astigmatism and loss of best-corrected visual acuity. Numerous risk factors for post refractive surgery ectasia have been determined to include high myopia, thin residual stromal beds (< 250 μm), patient age, preoperative corneal thickness < 500 μm, central corneal power > 47.00 diopters (D), and asymmetrical corneal steepening > 1.00 D. Recent studies conclude that preoperative irregular topography is one of the most important risk factors associated with eyes that develop ectasia after refractive surgery. However, post refractive surgery ectasia has been reported in the absence of these risk factors. Although useful as general clinical guidelines, these risk factors remain controversial. For example, several

studies have shown no increased risk of ectasia in eyes with thin corneas. Also, there are isolated case reports of ectasia in eyes with thicker residual stromal beds.

Topographically, post refractive surgery ectasia resembles keratoconus. The hallmarks are inferior steepening on the axial power map, as well as elevation abnormalities noted first posteriorly and later anteriorly. However, the presence of central flattening from myopic excimer laser surgery complicates the topographic interpretation.

Evidence increasingly suggests that post surgical ectasia is, in fact, not a separate entity but rather represents keratoconus that was not diagnosed or detected prior to refractive surgery. Therefore, the ability to detect and identify such eyes preoperatively is paramount.

Wang M, Kugler LJ. *Atlas and Clinical Reference Guide for Corneal Topography (pp 133-140)*. © 2014 SLACK Incorporated.

AXIAL CURVATURE: ANTERIOR

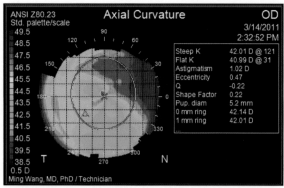

Figure 11-1. Atlas Placido-disk topography (Carl Zeiss Meditec) axial curvature map is from a patient diagnosed with post-LASIK ectasia. The asymmetric bent bow tie is the classic appearance of this condition and is indistinguishable from keratoconus, other than the keratometry (K) readings are much flatter. Note the K values are in the normal range, as the eye has been flattened with LASIK, thus offsetting the steepening caused from the ectasia.

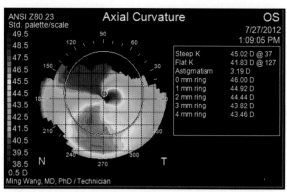

Figure 11-2. Axial curvature map shows asymmetric bow-tie pattern with inferior steepening. Patient history and flatter Ks are clues that this is post-LASIK ectasia rather than keratoconus.

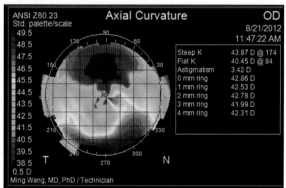

Figure 11-3. Axial curvature shows inferior steepening in the periphery of the cornea and a markedly flat area superiorly in the laser ablation zone.

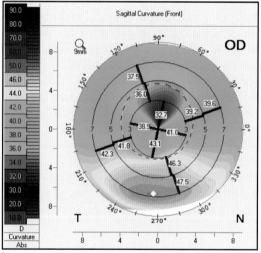

Figure 11-4. The flatter Ks and inferior steepening are consistent with post-laser-assisted in-situ keratomileusis (LASIK) ectasia.

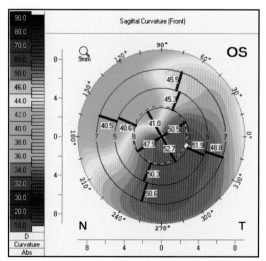

Figure 11-5. A severe case of post-LASIK ectasia with an approximately 12.00 D I-S difference (the difference between the inferior and superior curvature) is shown.

ANTERIOR ELEVATION

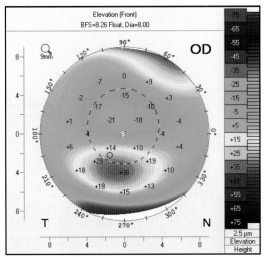

Figure 11-6. The anterior elevation in this map shows steepening of 36 µm. The superior adjacent flattening (blue) is the area of the laser ablation.

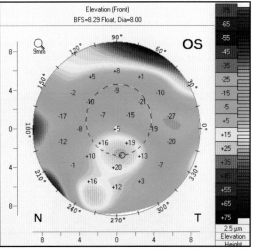

Figure 11-7. A strong asymmetry is noted in this cornea, and, without clinical correlation, it is difficult to be certain that this eye is post-LASIK.

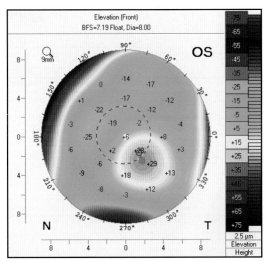

Figure 11-8. Typical pattern of central and superior flattening, contrasted with inferior elevation, is shown in this eye with post-LASIK ectasia.

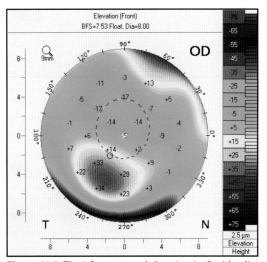

Figure 11-9. The inferotemporal elevation (red) with adjacent thinning (blue) is typical of an eye with an ectatic process.

POSTERIOR ELEVATION

As with other topographic maps, because post refractive surgery ectasia is thought to represent undiagnosed keratoconus and not a distinct condition, many of the topographic findings on posterior elevation maps are indistinguishable between the two diagnoses. Signs of post-LASIK ectasia are detected on the posterior elevation map prior to the other maps.

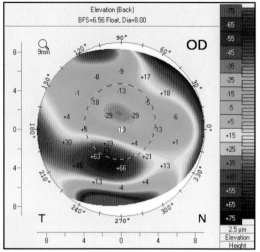

Figure 11-10. Posterior elevation map in this post-LASIK ectasia eye shows a markedly elevated area inferiorly.

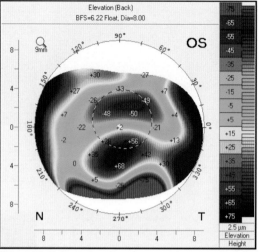

Figure 11-11. Posterior elevation map shows marked elevation of > 68 μm (dark red). The adjacent flattening (dark blue) contributes to a difference of more than 120 μm in the central area of the cornea.

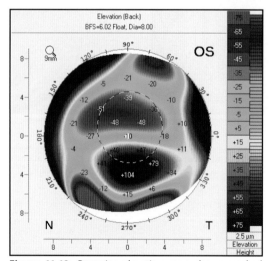

Figure 11-12. Posterior elevation map shows marked elevation of 104 μm. This patient was diagnosed with post-refractive surgery ectasia.

PACHYMETRIC MAPS

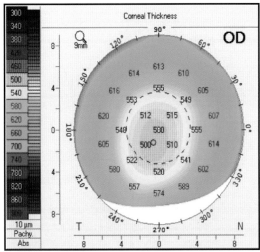

Figure 11-13. The thinnest point in a pachymetry map is typically decentered in ectatic corneas, such as in keratoconus and post-LASIK ectasia eyes.

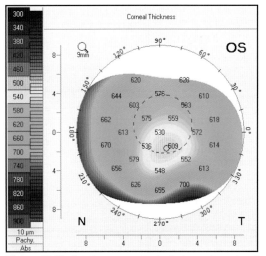

Figure 11-14. Ectatic corneas typically have decentered apexes, with thinning inferiorly as seen in the orange area of this pachymetry map.

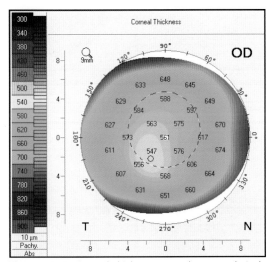

Figure 11-15. Corneal thickness map shows a relatively normal cornea with slight inferotemporal decentering of the thinnest area of the cornea (light green). The diagnosis of ectasia cannot be made from the pachymetric map alone, but it offers important clues.

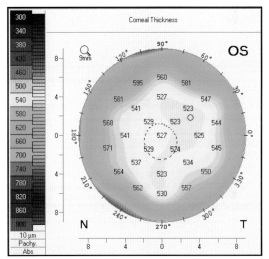

Figure 11-16. As noted in most maps showing corneal thickness, the thinnest area is typically in a circular, evenly distributed pattern. On observation of this corneal thickness map, the area in yellow and orange is asymmetric and unevenly distributed across the cornea, which is most likely due to a distorted cornea. This map alone could not lead to a diagnosis of ectasia, but an irregular thickness pattern is not typical after refractive surgery, thus it raises suspicion for further investigation.

FOUR-MAP REFRACTIVE VIEW

Figure 11-17. Ectasia refers to progressive thinning that produces irregular astigmatism, asymmetric steepening, and areas of abnormal elevation. In this 4-map refractive picture, the sagittal curvature map shows marked inferior steepening at 51.00 D, which results in irregular astigmatism. The corneal thickness map shows that the thinnest portion is 514 µm, within the range of normal for a post-LASIK eye. However, the anterior and posterior elevation maps are markedly abnormal and explain why there is such severe steepening and irregularity. Post surgical ectasia may be differentiated from keratoconus by the relatively flat K readings centrally on the axial power map, as well as the area of flattening on the anterior elevation map.

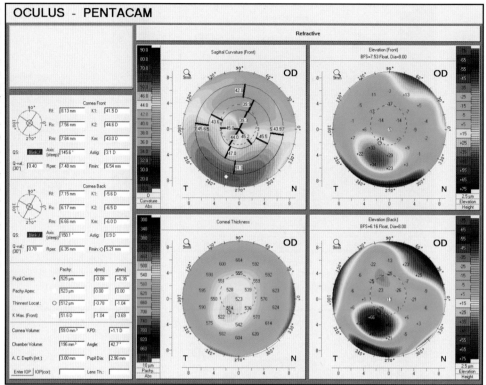

Figure 11-18. It can easily be determined from this combination of refractive maps that the patient has an irregular, asymmetric cornea with severe ectasia. Posterior elevation is more marked than the anterior elevation, which is typical of ectatic diseases, with the posterior portion of the cornea being affected first and thus more severely affected than the anterior portion. Without the patient's diagnosis of prior refractive surgery, this 4-map refractive picture may be confused with keratoconus, although the area of flattening superonasally on the anterior elevation map is an important clue.

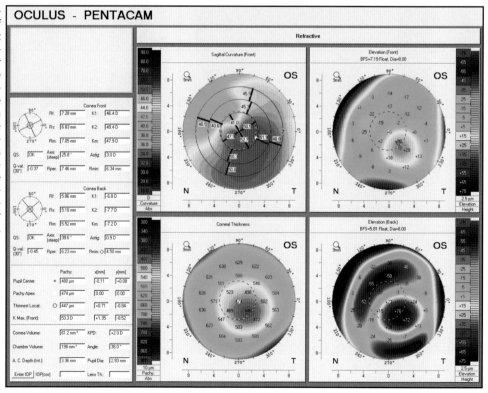

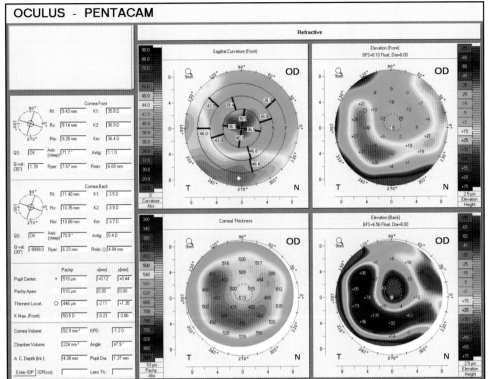

Figure 11-19. Four-map refractive picture demonstrates a patient who is ectatic after radial keratotomy (RK) surgery. Ectasia after RK is a very different condition than ectasia after excimer laser surgery. Typically, ectasia after RK is the result of gaping incisions. In this eye, the severely elevated areas inferiorly and nasally correspond to gaping astigmatic keratotomy and RK incisions. Interestingly, the central cornea overlying the small pupil is still flat and relatively symmetric.

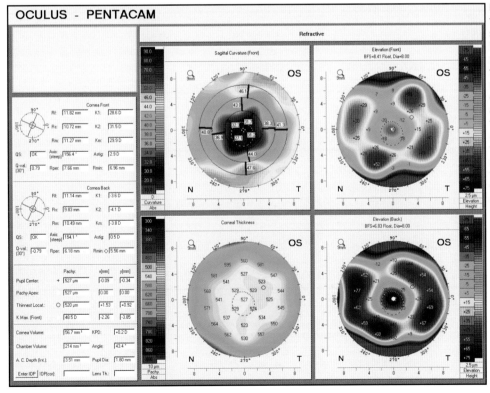

Figure 11-20. Collection of maps that shows a patient who had RK surgery years prior. The authors include these to demonstrate map examples that often are confused with ectasia; however, the patient probably does not have ectasia. The peripheral elevation abnormalities are consistent with the location of the RK incisions and represent anterior elevation of the cornea in those areas. There is severe flattening centrally, more so than was intended by the surgeon, which is the consequence of progressively gaping peripheral radial incisions.

Figure 11-21. Four-map refractive picture shows a classic representation of keratoconus. However, knowing the patient's history of previous refractive surgery indicates that this is a case of post refractive ectasia.

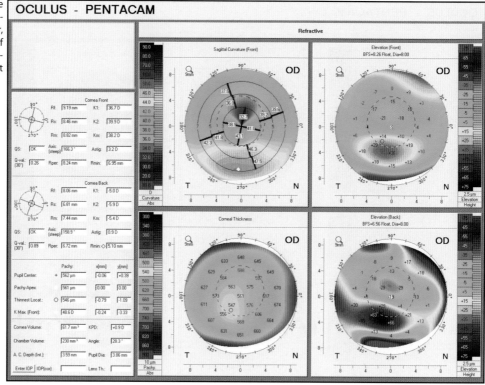

Epithelial Basement Membrane Dystrophy

Epithelial basement membrane dystrophy (EBMD), also known as map-dot-fingerprint dystrophy, Cogan's dystrophy, and anterior basement membrane dystrophy, is a noninfectious, noninflammatory disorder of the basement membrane of the epithelium. In general, the basement membrane becomes thickened and irregular. The condition is often bilateral, but it can have marked asymmetry in its presentation, resulting in a large difference between the 2 eyes.

Often first appearing in patients over 30 years old, initial presentation can be asymptomatic or as severe as transient blurred vision and painful recurrent erosions.

The thickened and irregular epithelium causes abnormally appearing topographic images that are often confused with other disorders. This chapter covers some of the common findings in these eyes.

Axial Curvature

The appearance of EBMD in axial curvature maps is variable. The hallmarks are irregular astigmatism with keratometry (K) values that vary dramatically. Such irregularity in K readings often leads to erroneous intraocular lens calculations at the time of cataract surgery in these patients. Abnormal topography is an important indication to proceed with caution when calculating intraocular lens power prior to cataract surgery.

Wang M, Kugler LJ. *Atlas and Clinical Reference Guide for Corneal Topography (pp 141-148).* © 2014 SLACK Incorporated.

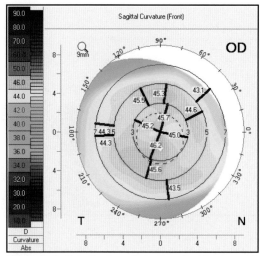

Figure 12-1. Note the irregular pattern in this map, with the suggestion of inferior steepening. This map may be confused with early keratoconus.

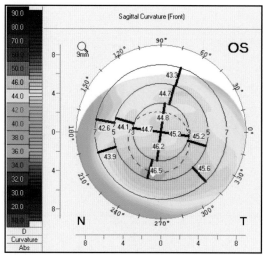

Figure 12-2. Example of EBMD that could easily be confused as keratoconus. One differentiating clue is the large degree of irregularity across the entire corneal surface, including the superior half of the cornea.

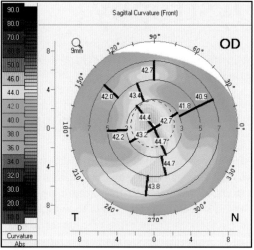

Figure 12-3. Central and inferior steepening in an eye with EBMD. Note that the thickening of the epithelium causes this picture and not actually a steepening of the corneal contour.

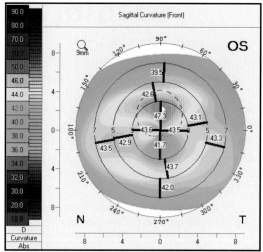

Figure 12-4. Irregularity of the epithelium causes the appearance of superior steepening and irregular astigmatism in this EBMD eye.

ANTERIOR CURVATURE

Anterior curvature maps are very useful in distinguishing EBMD from ectatic disorders.

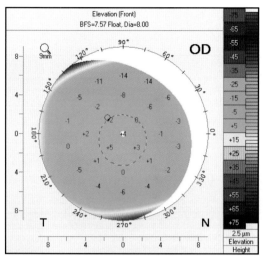

Figure 12-5. In this eye with severe EBMD, the anterior elevation map is normal.

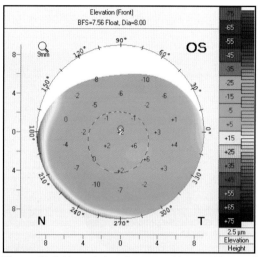

Figure 12-6. Normal elevation map with no evidence of an ectatic process.

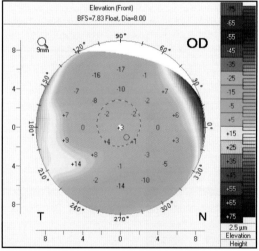

Figure 12-7. Normal elevation map in an eye with high with-the-rule astigmatism and EBMD.

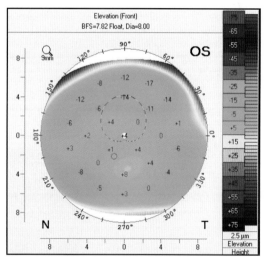

Figure 12-8. Note the suggestion of mild elevation inferiorly in this eye with severe EBMD. In this eye, the epithelial thickening is severe enough to cause a change in measured elevation. The next step in this eye would be to look at the posterior elevation map, which is likely to be normal for EBMD but abnormal for an ectatic condition.

POSTERIOR CURVATURE

Posterior curvature maps are generally normal in EBMD patients, as the abnormality in this disease is confined solely to the anterior surface epithelium. However, the posterior maps are prone to artifact due to the opacity often caused by epithelial clumping and scarring.

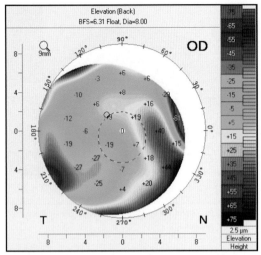

Figure 12-9. The appearance of this posterior elevation map is suggestive of artifact due to the irregular pattern of the elevation and its location nasally. This pattern is not consistent with keratoconus or ectasia, thus artifact must be considered.

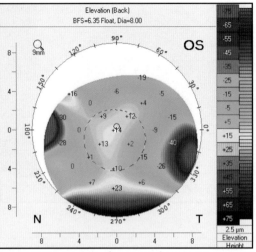

Figure 12-10. Example of an unusual-appearing posterior elevation map. The elevation noted centrally and in the far inferior periphery is not typical of that seen in keratoconus or ectasia.

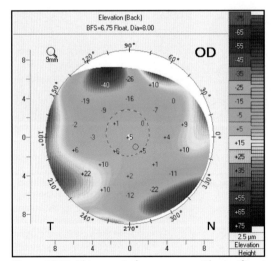

Figure 12-11. This map is from an eye with significant EMBD, but it is without scarring severe enough to cause artifact in the posterior elevation measurement.

PACYHMETRIC MAPS

Pacyhmetric maps in EBMD are generally normal, but if the thickening is severe enough to cause measureable changes in thickness, it may change the appearance of the map.

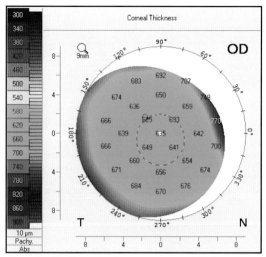

Figure 12-12. Example of a grossly normal thickness map, with the suggestion of some thickening in the central and superior midperiphery.

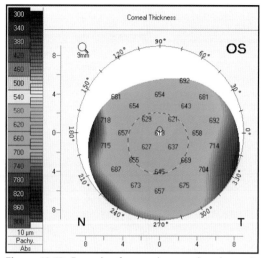

Figure 12-13. Example of a grossly normal pachymetric map in an eye with EBMD.

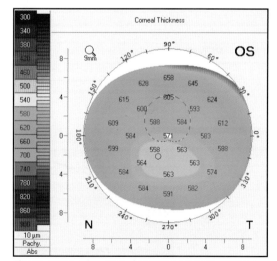

Figure 12-14. This map demonstrates how EBMD can emulate keratoconus. The epithelium in this cornea has thickened superiorly, where the thinnest point appears to be inferior. An important clue that this is likely not ectasia is the thick measurement of 558 µm at the thinnest point. In an eye with keratoconus or ectasia, the thinnest point would be much thinner than it is in this eye.

FOUR-MAP REFRACTIVE VIEW

Figure 12-15. Example of an eye with EBMD that was misdiagnosed as keratoconus. The axial power map is consistent with keratoconus and shows marked inferior steepening with an irregular bow-tie appearance. The anterior elevation and posterior elevation maps are normal, thus ruling out the diagnosis of ectasia. The pachymetric map reflects the thickening of the epithelium that has occurred superonasally, which caused the irregular appearance on the axial power map, as well as the deviation of the thinnest point on the pachymetric map.

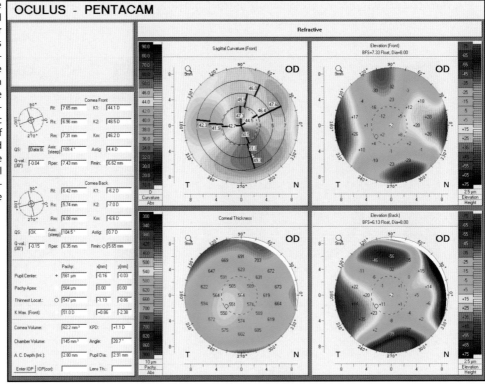

Figure 12-16. Example of EBMD causing the irregular astigmatism shown on this axial power map, but no change in the elevation maps is noted. The epithelial thickening superonasally in this eye has caused a shift in the thinnest point on the pachymetric map. As with all cases of possible ectasia or keratoconus, the elevation maps are essential in determining that this is not an eye with ectatic disease.

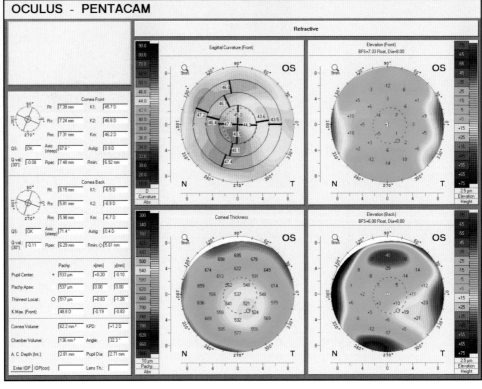

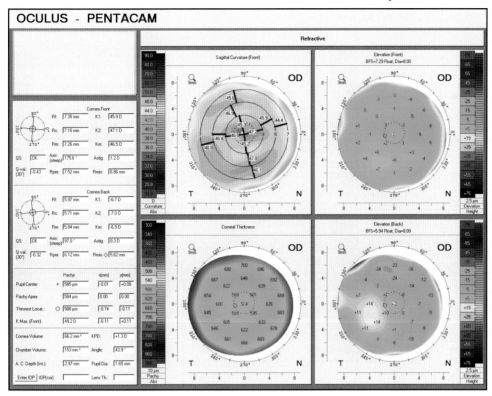

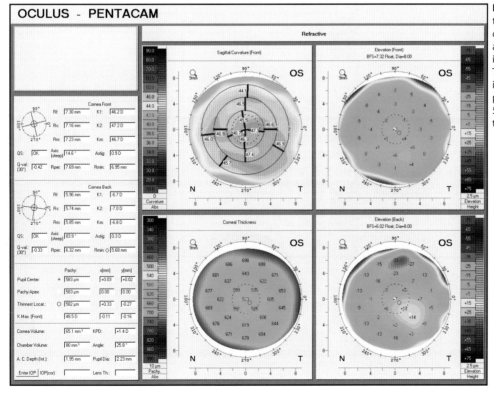

Figure 12-17. This is a complicated map that requires careful consideration before drawing any conclusions. The axial power map is severely irregular, with no discernible pattern. Such irregularity is the first clue that this eye has an epithelial problem, which could include EBMD or severe dry eye. The anterior elevation map is grossly normal, but it has a suggestion of an early elevation abnormality inferotemporally. The posterior elevation map has an area of abnormal elevation, which in this case is an artifact caused by EBMD scarring. The pachymetric map is normal, with no evidence of thinnest point displacement corresponding to the area of posterior elevation. Because there is no correlation between the anterior elevation, posterior elevation, and pachymetric maps in this eye, we know it does not have keratoconus or ectasia. The irregularity on the axial power map helps to confirm the diagnosis of an epithelial problem, which in this case is EBMD. On resolution of the epithelial irregularity, the posterior elevation map would likely normalize.

Figure 12-18. Example of EBMD that caused an irregular anterior corneal surface, leading to irregular astigmatism and artifact abnormality in the posterior elevation map. The pachymetric map is useful here in distinguishing from an ectatic process, as the thinnest point is 595 µm and not corresponding to the area of posterior elevation.

Figure 12-19. Although the posterior elevation abnormality is suspicious for an early ectatic process, careful examination of the other 3 maps suggests this is not a case of keratoconus or ectasia. The axial power map has an irregular pattern that is not consistent with an ectatic disorder. The axial power map is normal. The pachymetric map shows a thinnest point of 575 µm, which is not consistent with corneal thinning. This constellation of findings leads to the diagnosis of an epithelial disorder, which in this case is EBMD. The abnormality in the posterior elevation map is likely an artifact from the opacities caused by EBMD.

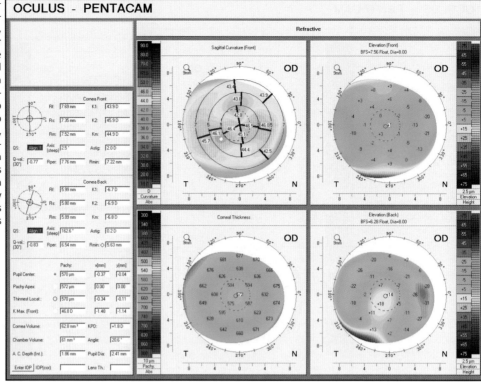

Figure 12-20. Example of EBMD, which is similar to that presented in Figure 12-19. The axial power map shows a surface with marked irregular astigmatism. The anterior elevation map is normal without evidence of ectasia. The posterior elevation map has an area of increased elevation, but it does not correspond with the other 3 maps. The thickness map measures 552 µm at the thinnest point, which is not consistent with ectasia.

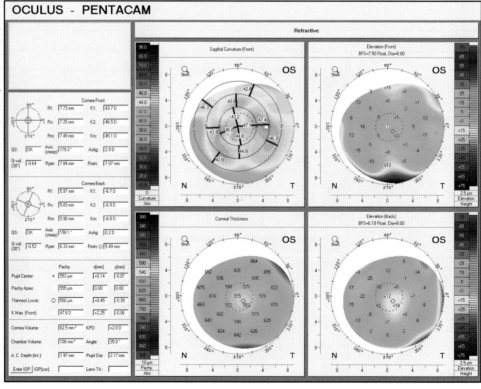

Fuchs' Endothelial Dystrophy

As Fuchs' dystrophy progresses and the cornea becomes more edematous, many subtle topographic findings are seen, which are discussed in this chapter.

AXIAL CURVATURE

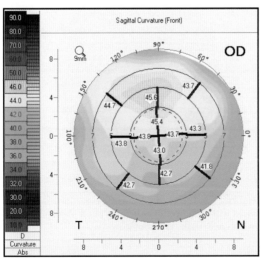

Figure 13-1. Superior steepening is a rare finding on topography, and it almost never is the result of an ectatic process. Therefore, the diagnosis of Fuchs' dystrophy should always be considered when encountering a map with this appearance.

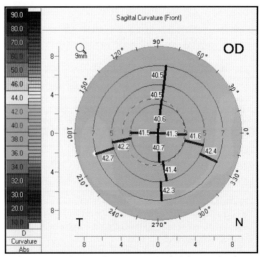

Figure 13-2. This eye has severe Fuchs' dystrophy, but it has a completely normal axial power map.

Wang M, Kugler LJ. *Atlas and Clinical Reference Guide for Corneal Topography* (pp 149-156). © 2014 SLACK Incorporated.

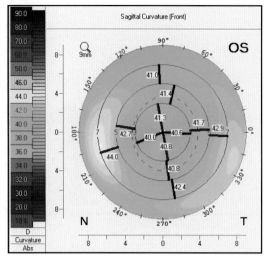

Figure 13-3. This Fuchs' eye has mild central irregularity, with some steepening in the far nasal periphery as a result of the central thickening.

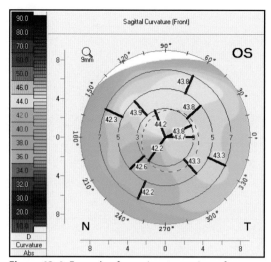

Figure 13-4. Example of superior steepening, often seen in eyes with Fuchs' dystrophy.

ANTERIOR CURVATURE

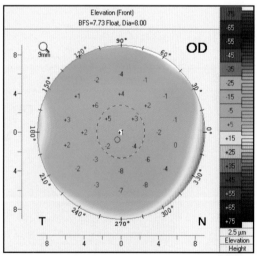

Figure 13-5. Example shows an area of mild elevation in the superior midperiphery. Superior elevation is not consistent with an ectatic process, but it can be seen in eyes with Fuchs' dystrophy.

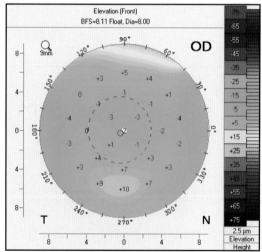

Figure 13-6. The inferior increased elevation may be confused with keratoconus or ectasia, but it may also be seen in eyes with Fuchs' dystrophy.

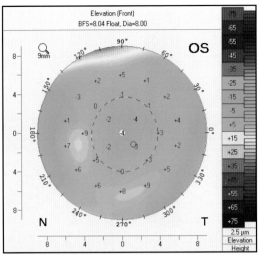

Figure 13-7. This eye demonstrates a diffuse elevation in the midperiphery in a circumferential pattern. This pattern is consistent, although it is not patognomonic for Fuchs' disease.

POSTERIOR CURVATURE

Because Fuchs' disease causes edema throughout the corneal stroma in an irregular distribution, virtually any pattern may be seen on a posterior elevation map.

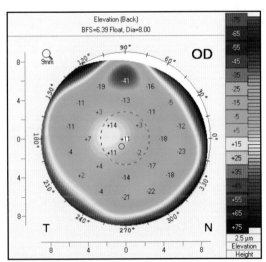

Figure 13-8. Edema in this cornea is concentrated in the mid to far periphery, causing a relative increase in elevation near the center.

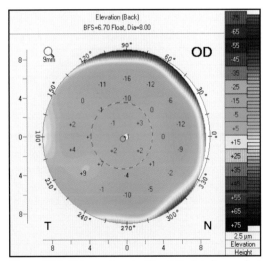

Figure 13-9. This eye has significant Fuchs' disease, but because the edema is symmetric throughout the cornea, there are no areas of relative elevation abnormality.

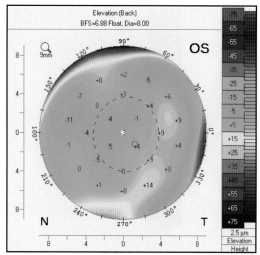

Figure 13-10. Irregular distribution of corneal edema is causing areas of relative elevation differences in the mid-periphery of this eye with Fuchs' dystrophy.

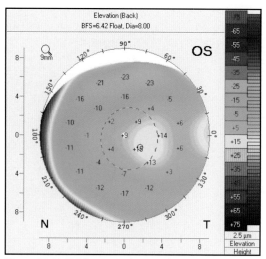

Figure 13-11. Thickening in the periphery causes a relative elevation centrally.

PACHYMETRIC MAPS

Because the hallmark of Fuchs' dystrophy is corneal edema, the pachymetric map in eyes with this disease shows diffuse corneal edema with increased thickness.

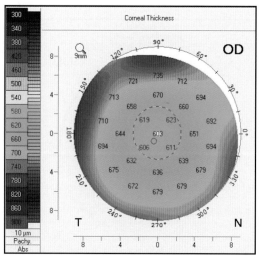

Figure 13-12. Note the high corneal thickness measurements both centrally and peripherally.

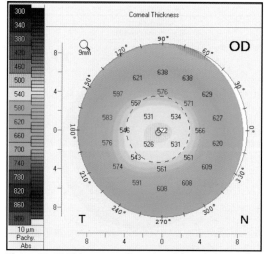

Figure 13-13. This map confirms that although this eye has clinical signs of Fuchs' dystrophy, the disease has not yet caused corneal edema.

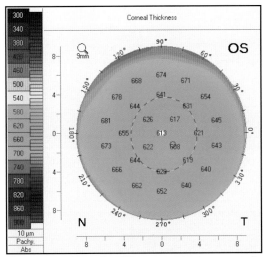

Figure 13-14. Note the diffuse corneal edema centrally and peripherally in this eye with significant Fuchs' disease.

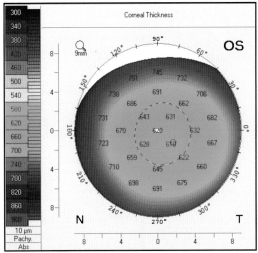

Figure 13-15. Pachymetric maps in eyes with Fuchs' are often blue in color due to the elevated thickness in the periphery.

FOUR-MAP REFRACTIVE VIEW

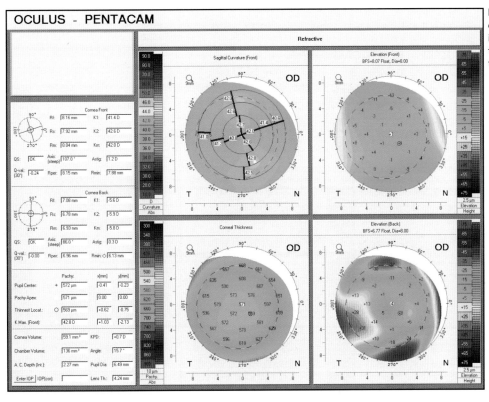

Figure 13-16. Clues to Fuchs' disease in this eye include nonspecific irregularity in the posterior elevation map, a normal anterior elevation map, and diffuse thickening.

Figure 13-17. Diffuse thickening is the primary finding in this set of maps. Nonspecific irregularity of the posterior elevation is noted, which is not consistent with an ectatic process.

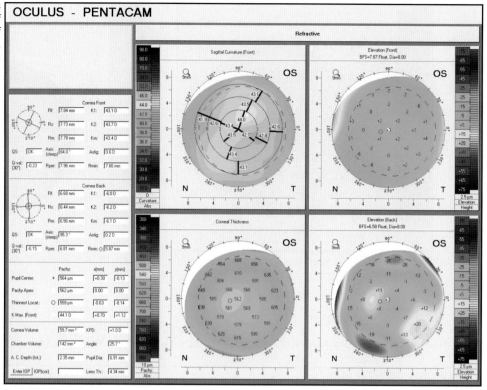

Figure 13-18. The steep inferior periphery on axial power map is suggestive of pellucid marginal degeneration; however, the other maps rule out this diagnosis. Note there is no correlation between the anterior and posterior elevation maps, thus there is no suggestion of an ectatic process. The pachymetric map has thickening in an irregular pattern more inferiorly than superiorly. This thickening is causing the irregular pattern seen on the axial power maps.

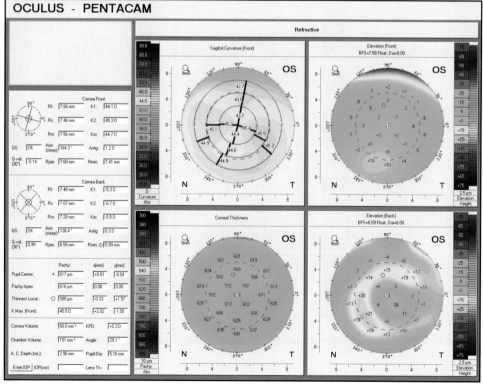

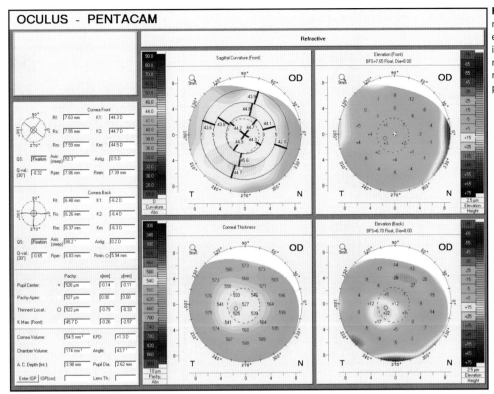

Figure 13-19. Without clinical correlation, this eye may be considered at risk for keratoconus. One important clue that the diagnosis is not keratoconus is the lack of inferior displacement of the thinnest point.

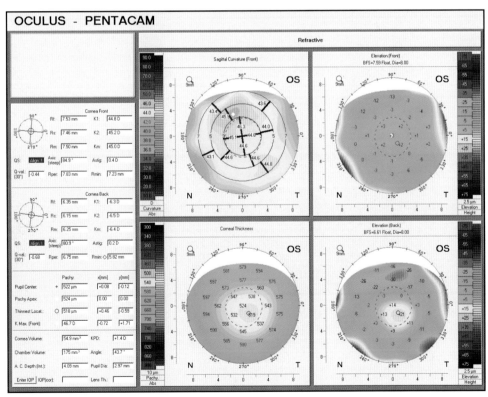

Figure 13-20. Superior steepening and an irregular posterior elevation map are consistent with Fuchs' dystrophy. Other considerations would be epithelial disease or dry eye.

Figure 13-21. Example of clinically significant Fuchs' disease, with mild posterior elevation irregularity and diffusely elevated corneal thickness.

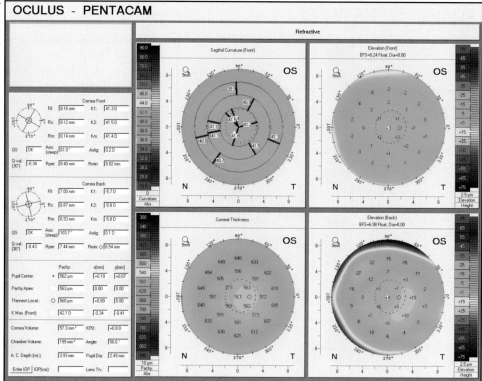

Bibliography

Belin MW, Khachikian SS. Elevation based topography: screening for refractive surgery. *Highlights of Ophthalmology.* 2008.

Binder PS. Risk factors for ectasia after LASIK. *J Cataract Refract Surg.* 2008;34(12):2010-2011.

Colin J, Touboul D. Algorithm for management of post-laser ectasia. *Cataract and Refractive Surgery Today Europe.* April;2010:36-38.

Donnenfeld ED, Randleman JB, Slade SG, Trattler WB. Refractive surgery on a thin cornea. *Cataract and Refractive Surgery Today.* May;2009.

Espandar L, Meyer J. Keratoconus: overview and update on treatment. *Middle East Afr J Ophthalmol.* 2010;17(1):15-20.

Eye Bank Association of America. *Eye Banking Statistical Report.* Washington, DC: Eye Bank Association of America; 2006.

Hardten DR, Gosavi VV. Point/counterpoint: refractive surgery in a keratoconus suspect. *Cataract and Refractive Surgery Today.* October;2006:66-71.

Hersh PS, Greenstein SA, Fry KL. Corneal collagen crosslinking for keratoconus and corneal ectasia: one-year results. *J Cataract Refract Surg.* 2011;37(1):149-160.

Hersch P. Managing post-LASIK ectasia. *Refractive Eyecare.* 2009;13(8):21-23.

Karmel M. The thick and thin of ectasia. *EyeNet Magazine.* January;2008.

Leibowitz HM, Waring GO III. *Corneal Disorders: Clinical Diagnosis and Management.* 2nd ed. Philadelphia, PA: WB Saunders; 1998.

Lipner M. Cutting to the truth about corneal ectasia. *EyeWorld.* January;2003.

McMahon TT, Szcotka-Flynn L, Barr JT, et al; CLEK Study Group. A new method for grading the severity of keratoconus: the Keratoconus Severity Score (KSS). *Cornea.* 2006;25(7):794-800.

Nordan LT. Forme fruste ectasia. *Cataract and Refractive Surgery Today.* September;2007:23-25.

Nordan LT, Trattler WB. Point/counterpoint: is corneal thickness a risk factor for post-LASIK ectasia? *Cataract and Refractive Surgery Today.* September;2007:58-64.

Rabinowitz YS. Diagnosing keratoconus and patients at risk. *Cataract and Refractive Surgery Today.* May;2007:85-87.

Rabinowitz YS. Keratoconus. *Surv Ophthalmol.* 1998;42(4):297-319.

Raiskup-Wolf F, Hoyer A, Spoerl E, Pillunat LE. Collagen crosslinking with riboflavin and ultraviolet-A light in keratoconus: long-term results. *J Cataract Refract Surg.* 2008;34(5):796-801.

Slade SG, Trattler WB, Woodhams T. Classifying keratoconus. *Cataract and Refractive Surgery Today.* August;2006:74-76.

Tasman WS, Jaeger EA. *The Wills Eye Hospital Atlas of Clinical Ophthalmology.* Philadelphia, PA: Lippincott Williams & Wilkins; 1996.

Trattler WB. Known risk factors for ectasia. *Cataract and Refractive Surgery Today.* October;2005:109-113.

Wang M, ed. Corneal Topography: *A Guide for Clinical Application in the Wavefront Era.* 2nd ed. Thorofare, NJ: SLACK Incorporated; 2012.

Weissman BA, Yeung KK. Keratoconus. Medscape Reference Web site. http://Emedicine.medscape.com/article/1194693-overview. Accessed February 12, 2010.

Woodward MA, Randleman JB, Russell B, Lynn MJ, Ward MA, Stulting RD. Visual rehabilitation and outcomes for ectasia after corneal refractive surgery. *J Cataract Refract Surg.* 2008;34(3):383-388.

Yeung KK, Weissman BA. 15th annual comanagement report: an introduction to corneal collagen cross-linking. *Review of Optometry.* 2010;147(3):90-95.

Financial Disclosures

Dr. Helen Boerman is a speaker for Allergan and Bausch & Lomb.

Dr. Lance J. Kugler has no financial or proprietary interest in the materials presented herein.

Dr. Linda A. Morgan has no financial or proprietary interest in the materials presented herein.

Dr. Ming Wang has no financial or proprietary interest in the materials presented herein.

Index